INDEXING MANAGED CARE

INDEXING MANAGED CARE

Benchmarking Strategies for Assessing Managed Care Penetration in Your Market

DENNIS J. PATTERSON

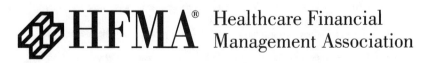 **HFMA**® Healthcare Financial Management Association

McGraw-Hill

New York   San Francisco   Washington, D.C.   Auckland   Bogotá
Caracas   Lisbon   London   Madrid   Mexico City   Milan
Montreal   New Delhi   San Juan   Singapore
Sydney   Tokyo   Toronto

Library of Congress Cataloging-in-Publication Data
Patterson, Dennis J.
   Indexing managed care : benchmarking strategies for assessing managed care penetration
in your market / Dennis J. Patterson.
     p.   cm.
   Includes bibliographical references and index.
   Includes bibliographical references and index.
   ISBN 0-7863-1067-7 (alk. paper)
   1. Managed care plans (Medical care)   I. Title.
   [DNLM: 1. Managed Care Programs—organization & administration—United States.
2. Managed Care Programs—utilization—United States. W 130 AA1 P2i 1997]
RA413.P38   1997
362.1′04258—dc21
DNLM/DLC
for Library of Congress   97-29562
                                                CIP

McGraw-Hill

*A Division of The **McGraw·Hill** Companies*

1 2 3 4 5 6 7 8 9 0 BKM / BKM 9 0 9 8 7

ISBN 0–7863–1067–7

Printed and bound by Book-Mart Press, Inc.

This publication is designed to provide accurate and authoritative information in regard to the subject matter covered. It is sold with the understanding that neither the author nor the publisher is en-
gaged in rendering legal, accounting, or other professional service. If legal advice or other expert
assistance is required, the services of a competent professional person should be sought.

     —From a Declaration of Principles jointly adopted by a Committee of the American
      Bar Association and a Committee of Publishers.

McGraw-Hill books are available at special quantity discounts to use as premiums and sales promo-
tions, or for use in corporate training programs. For more information, please write to the Director
of Sales, McGraw-Hill, 11 West 19th Street, New York, NY 10011.
Or contact your local bookstore.

This book is dedicated to Susan, Valerie, and Christina for their love and support.

PREFACE

That managed care will transform American healthcare is by now a reality or an impending certainty in virtually every local market. But providers and payors are clamoring to understand precisely how this revolution will effect their marketplaces and how they can best transform their organizations to embrace managed-care's manifold challenges and promises. Managed Care Indexing is designed to help healthcare organizations determine, in rather objective terms, their current states and future prospects. Together, dear reader, we will consider how to interpret and assimilate complex market information, how to understand the shifting managed-care landscape at a glance, and how to craft a prudent, responsive strategy.

The germ of this book was planted in the summer of 1993, when two old friends met at a Los Angeles airport restaurant to reminisce about their early days in Canadian healthcare and to discuss the future of healthcare in the United States. The topic of the day: Is there some meaningful and accurate way to measure the presence of managed care? The two friends were your author, just nicely taking the consulting helm for FHP, then California's fourth largest HMO, and Dr. Ian Morrison, President of The Institute For The Future, a renowned Bay Area think tank. Ian and I go back to our very first jobs at large teaching hospitals affiliated with the University of British Columbia. Over the years we have maintained our friendship and spoken of so many, many things. But the seemingly straightforward question we had decided to tackle over lunch looked more and more like the crux of a very important matter.

Can one actually measure the market penetration of managed care, not by counting how many people are enrolled in health maintenance or preferred provider organizations but, rather, by exploring what types of techniques the market's payors and providers are using? Could marketplaces then be rated on a scale from managed care "lite" to managed care "heavy"? To what good work might healthcare strategists put such a rating system?

ENTER THE INDEX

We envisioned a tool that would be readily distinguishable from other managed-care outlooks and gauges in its focus and practicality, one that would go well beyond merely tracking HMO penetration rates to examine the aggregate forces at work in a dynamic, emerging managed-care market. Together, these forces would paint a vivid picture of precisely how managed care changes a local healthcare community. Properly constructed and interpreted, the resulting change model would be utterly comprehensive.

Forging the tool proved to be a more demanding task than we had anticipated. A more elegant instrument always poses richer design problems. What we and our colleagues wanted was a handy index whose purpose would not be to prove how good or how cheap or even how effective managed care was but, instead, to measure how much managed-care activity was actually occurring in today's marketplace.

But one must define clearly what one endeavors to quantify wholly. Putting that first thing first, we had to acknowledge that we had only been pretending to know what managed care really *is*. Now, some 4 years later, everyone heartily agrees that managed care has arrived, but still no one has defined it succinctly to my satisfaction. In the course of assembling these writings, I interviewed some of managed care's bona fide movers and shakers, such as leading executives of sophisticated payor organizations, integrated providers, and physician groups—and not one of them could briefly define managed care without due hesitation, caveat, or apology. This should be no embarrassment to any of us, because no single definition suffices.

Managed care is the proverbial elephant described by five blindfolded men: individual perspectives border on the absurd, and the composite sketch portrays a beast far more marvelous or horrific than humdrum reality. So do not rely on eyewitness reports. You had better get to know the creature yourself now that it has come over to play in your backyard.

Several respectable bodies today claim to measure managed care. InterStudy and the American Association of Health Plans measure the number of enrollees in health maintenance organizations. The National Committee for Quality Assurance and the National Research Corporation both measure performance and consumer satisfaction with health plans. Employee Benefit Research Institute (EBRI) and Bureau of Labor (BOL) measure insurance and employee benefits. And the American Medical

Association, the American Hospital Association, and the Physician Management Association measure what their respective members care about. None of these measures adequately defines managed care, much less quantifies managed care presence in any objective or comprehensive manner. Nobody is getting at the key interfaces of managed care. Precisely what actions constitute the practice of managed healthcare?

After considerable research and brainstorming, the Institute For The Future found that basic managed-care activities in certain corners of the marketplace were influencing the behavior of virtually every other player in the system. Thus, the stated goals of our Managed-Care Index were to measure this activity by studying five highly influential groups and the techniques they were applying to effect or deflect the behavior of others. The groups studied include both healthcare system users (enrollees and patients) and providers (doctors, hospitals, and pharmacies). Again, any one of these perspectives alone cannot tell the whole story, so the Index employs data-gathering and analytic techniques that present these market forces in aggregate.

Like managed care itself, the index is still in painful transition. Further studies are under way to incorporate the index's underlying elements into even more powerful tools.

A CERTAIN FLAIR

A core challenge in developing the Managed-Care index was to paint targets on moving objects. We sought to report managed care's growth in different markets progressing at different speeds, and we learned to battle against the seeming futility of this exercise with levity. We made our biggest conceptual breakthroughs with humor and clever turns of phrase. Several provocative themes arose during our initial research, at speeches and conferences Ian and I have conducted, and from sundry items that cropped up in the news and in the literature.

Many major hospital systems, for instance, are struggling to capture hospital beds to make themselves managed-care ready, but just as surely they are readying themselves for extinction. We call it the *Last Waltz of the Dinosaurs*. Managed-care *lite* had all the right connotations, we felt, to describe the less-filling-tastes-great HMO and PPO products so many indemnity insurance companies are rolling out, then claiming great success, without so much as bothering to employ a single managed-care technique. We also took to calling this phenomenon *Indemnity in Drag*.

Finally, through interviews I conducted with recognized leaders in managed-care organizations, hospital systems, and physician systems across the nation, it became clear to me that many of the underlying assumptions creating organized delivery systems, physician groups, independent practice associations, and new insurance products are indeed just interim steps toward the real healthcare system of the future. The *Managed-Care Pinwheel* introduced in Chapter 3, and used as a unifying motif throughout the book, portrays the future model I hold constantly in mind. The pinwheel might just as easily have been coined a turbine or a vortex or some such fancy term more liable to wow the industry, forgive the touch of whimsy.

The basic assumption behind the managed-care pinwheel is that capital sharing among system entities, merely for the sake of capturing one another's businesses, will not create the financing and delivery model we should desire. Only the free exchange of intellectual capital through advanced information technology and case management techniques, all with a sharp eye toward better health outcomes, will keep managed care moving in the right direction. (You may wish to count along as I repeat the preceding kernel of wisdom throughout this book.) Once devised and refined, my little pinwheel figure made the folly of strong central control and ownership all too clear. The current wave of hospitals, physicians, and insurance companies using their precious capital dollars to acquire and operate other parts of the system does not, in my view, make a lot of sense.

As a good friend of mine, Dr. Jim Austin, a former medical director for several Southern California managed-care entities, puts it: "Saying that you can own different parts of the healthcare system is like saying you own your children."

OUR DESIGN

As its section headings indicate, this book aims to help you understand today's managed-care landscape, measure managed-care presence in your marketplace, pilot your organization's managed-care transformation, and look ahead to the next industry revolution.

Readers will first explore the very basics of contemporary managed care, principles everyone thinks they know but so few actually understand or put into daily practice. The managed-care fundamentals we discuss in Chapter 1 include managing health, defining and insuring covered populations, evolving from a sickness treatment to a health concept of care delivery and financing, and managing clinical and business risk at once by providing the right care, in the right setting, and at the lowest cost.

In Chapter 2 we explain how the healthcare community today must adapt to three prevailing trends: (1) hospitals, through integration and the incessant shifting of traditional acute care into alternative settings, are fast becoming "centers of health" rather than sickness care facilities; (2) acute care institutions are downsizing constantly and becoming more expense-intensive care units; and (3) vacated acute care spaces are being filled by ambulatory care, skilled nursing, extended care, and health diagnostic centers. This chapter examines how providers, payors, and physicians, in unprecedented and often troublesome collaborations, are responding to these trends. It further identifies the potential beneficiaries and casualties of such powerful forces for change.

Chapter 3 introduces the Managed-Care Pinwheel, in all its mystery and splendor. Enjoy.

Next, in Chapter 4, we consider the viewpoints, activities, and dispositions that will shape the future of managed care. The conversations we eavesdrop upon here have been assembled from my travels and personal meetings with some of managed care's luminaries and voices of authority.

Chapter 5 presents the chief components of the Managed-Care Index and establishes its conceptual framework. In essence, the Index tracks the telltale signs of managed care evolution (financial incentives, micromanagement, integration of medicine, provider panel restrictions, and acceptance) exhibited by all major healthcare system participants, both users (patients, enrollees) and providers (physicians, hospitals, pharmacies). Chapter 5 then asks you to survey your own healthcare marketplace at-a-glance. Successful healthcare strategists have long been aware that there is no substitute for an intimate knowledge of one's own covered population and local market. Such knowledge never comes easy. A dynamic tool and a living discipline for establishing such a knowledge base, the Index embraces "managed care" as an umbrella term that encompasses all the participants and component forces introduced in Chapters 3 and 4. Such forces can be quantified, weighted, combined, and then meaningfully compared to historical and national data. The resulting index is a highly useful tool for measuring any market's level of managed-care penetration and the pace and momentum of ongoing change. Here readers will learn how the Managed-Care Index can be used to construct a vivid model of their own future marketplace.

Unlike other, conventional interpretations of market evolution, the Index quantifies managed care presence using a rigorous scoring system and comparative databases. Chapter 6 presents some survey instruments and other techniques used to compile raw information and explains the Index's sophisticated but practical system of scales and weights, through which essential survey, statistical, comparative, and empirical data are converted to an overall score of managed care presence. The scaled and weighted indicators discussed here include patient-managed-care incentives, enrollee provider panel restrictions, physician financial incentives, micromanagement of physicians, physician integration of practice setting, physician referral restrictions, hospital financial incentives, hospital micromanagement, hospital integration of medicine, micromanagement of pharmaceuticals, patient acceptance, and physician acceptance.

A guide to interpreting and applying the information produced through managed-care indexing, Chapter 7 dispenses practical advice regarding how all components of a healthcare market, providers and payors together, can begin the stepwise journey from managed care "lite" to managed care "heavy." Readers will learn how to put the Managed-Care Index to work as a reliable benchmarking tool and a solid planning base.

The transformation toward managed care requires constant tending. Chapter 8 explores proven methods that have guided successful managed-care organizations through the change process. Readers will specifically consider the benefits of establishing an Office of Managed Care Development, an executive enterprise created solely to direct the stepwise progress of the burgeoning managed-care organization.

What might our healthcare system look like once managed care sweeps the union? What forces might accompany or usurp the marketplace reforms under way today? In Chapter 9, reconnaissance reports from today's pioneering markets will give readers a glimpse into the future of managed care, and beyond.

I do so fervently hope that *Managed-Care Indexing* will serve those of you who, like me, deal day in and day out with an American health system in crisis. Healthcare organizations are being drawn, some dragged kicking and screaming, into sophisticated managed-care arrangements. In these pages I aspire to help physician, hospital, and managed-care executives judge the pace and extent of the most relevant changes in their markets, while arming them with the knowledge to formulate clear strategies not only to cope but to prosper in the 21st century.

As I have grown fond of saying: I will tell you about the present; if it sounds like the future, you may be living in the past.

ACKNOWLEDGEMENTS

Rarely is a book, or any major endeavor, the work of a lone individual. Let me take this opportunity to mention several people who made *Managed-Care Indexing* possible.

First and foremost, Dr. Ian Morrison, friend and colleague, who created the substance behind the Managed-Care Index. Portions of Chapters 5 and 6, as well as Appendix B, are presented here with kind permission of Dr. Morrison and The Institute for the Future.

An impressive cast of very busy people gave generously of their time to meet with me and inform my understanding of managed care today. Because each perspective was of such vital importance to the finished product, I list the contributors in alphabetical order: Laurence Abramson, President, SelectCare Health Plans, and Senior Vice President, Business Development, Peace Health; Terry Hartshorn, President and Chief Executive Officer, UniHealth; Janice James, Chief Financial Officer, Peace Health; Jack Kasten, JD, MPH, Professor, Department of Health Policy and Management, Harvard School of Public Health; Richard B. Lanman, MD, Founder and Chief Executive Officer, Adesso Specialty Services Organization; David M. Lawrance, MD, Chairman and Chief Executive Officer, Kaiser Foundation Health Plans; Kent Marquardt, Senior Vice President, Finance, MedPartners; Walter McNerney, Professor, Health Services Management, J. L. Kellogg Graduate School of Management, Northwestern University; and William A. Snow, PhD, Director of International Programs, California School of Professional Psychology.

Special thanks to my two secretaries, Suzann Reynolds and Mary O'Brien, who translated my ramblings into typescript.

Finally, I wish to acknowledge the three people who have most influenced my career in health administration: Edmund Lawler, who guided me into hospital administration; David Shade, who rescued me into the world of consulting; and Robert Kelly, whose belief in my abilities stretched me into the world of international consulting.

CONTENTS

1

Managed-Care Fundamentals

Through years of overuse and careless misuse, *managed care* has become perhaps the most seriously misunderstood term in the business lexicon. We have asked two common, tired words to do an impossibly big job. Try grasping firmly the perpetual motion of healthcare, an utterly complex human endeavor that is at once a hard science and a healing art, a caring tradition and a competitive business. Try describing concisely the lofty philosophies and intricate mechanisms by which a third of our nation's economy will someday operate. Try imagining an embryonic theory of healthcare financing and delivery that has been crowned the once and future king of a bold new marketplace.

Well, try we must, with two plain words to guide us. You are about to formulate your own personal working definition of managed care by devouring (or so a humble author may wish) this book-length elaboration upon the contemporary principles, techniques, and market dynamics of American healthcare.

First we will briefly explore the very basics of managed care—principles and techniques everyone thinks they know but so few actually understand or put into daily practice. The higher managed-care principles include prepayment, impanelment, and membership; managing health; defining and insuring populations; controlling risk; processing information;

and managing outcomes. The basic techniques that serve these higher principles include education, screening, and prevention; case management; utilization review and management; clinical pathways; continuous quality improvement; organizational change management; incentive systems; population study; and actuarial analysis.

Later chapters explore the market activities that have surrounded the introduction of managed-care principles and techniques and the forces that will ultimately shape the future of American healthcare. Together these writings aspire to build an uncommonly grand and accurate portrait of what we far too loosely call managed care.

MANAGED CARE VERY NEARLY DEFINED

In the eyes of most objective scholars and industry observers, the United States' healthcare financing and delivery system today is too fragmented, too expensive, and too ineffective against the worst enemies of our good health. How can we do better? Managed care is the short answer that begs this long-standing question.

We can do better by managing care itself, instead of just policing resources, finances, or numbers. We can do a much better job of determining when and where our rich variety of clinical disciplines can provide the most effective diagnoses, treatments, and therapies. Better yet, we can foster the healthy behaviors that prevent illness. Focusing sharply on best demonstrated practices and processes, we can intervene as intelligently and as early as possible, whenever possible, to stop healthy people from becoming ill, stop illnesses from becoming chronic ailments, and stop chronic ailments from becoming unduly harsh or premature threats to life. Should such preventions fail, as we know they often do, a finely tuned backup system (that is, our traditional acute care system) must be ever ready to spring into action to restore health as completely and efficiently as possible.

Our general definition could well end here, with a new zeal for prevention and a thorough tune-up of traditional clinical processes. If only it were that simple. We must explore the many facets of managed care to fully appreciate why this revolutionary healthcare concept so stubbornly defies brief explanation.

Three Easy Pieces

The term *managed care* attaches a perfectly fine adjective to a perfectly fine noun, but I prefer to think of it as an even stronger compound of the two active verbs: *to manage* and *to care.* You see, I am keen on balancing healthcare's business, clinical, and human/social agendas on this single fulcrum.

My definition of managed care therefore begins by dividing the whole matter into three pieces. Managed care comprises the following:

1. Higher Principles—the confluence of brilliant ideas by which we can envision a brighter healthcare future and embark upon the journey toward total population health management;

2. Basic Techniques—the set of proven tools by which we can better orchestrate all of our essential healthcare resources (people, technologies, and information) to preserve or improve health; and

3. Market Forces—the whirlwind of activity by which our healthcare system must weather significant change and somehow realign itself for the managed care future.

These three pieces must be fully understood separately before they can be meaningfully reassembled, much like an organist learns the right hand part, then the left hand, and finally the bass pedal line before trying to play all three together.

From here, any number of distinct viewpoints and partially acceptable definitions can take wing. No doubt we are defining managed care as we go along, to suit our own best interests. The words managed care must prove every bit as flexible as the systems, organizations, and minds through which managed care will become not just words but an everyday practice in every marketplace. Soon, though, our lively discourse must resolve into a commonly understandable definition, even if that definition cannot be uttered in a single breath by any solitary observer.

Many Viewpoints to Consider

Ask five people what managed care means and you will get five different answers, none right, none wrong. The relevant definition of managed care varies a great deal between industry sectors and among the disciplines and individuals within any given sector. A poor general definition would present an unsatisfying average of all viewpoints; a better definition, I think, would let each distinct viewpoint stand or fall on its own merits.

To begin with one popular view, chosen almost completely at random, managed care may accurately be described as a market-based system of care that strictly assigns accountabilities for both clinical and economic results to the professionals who wield the most control over those results. Every payor, medical group, and provider organization participating in the managed-care system has to live up to its respective accountabilities, good or bad. Because all segments of the healthcare system bear considerable new risk and feel more and more economic and competitive pressure, many people highlight these aspects in their definition of managed care.

Most often, it seems, careful observers define managed care via a process of elimination, one by one enumerating all the things managed care most certainly is not. Many people feel that the term managed care has been watered down and, in everyday practice and speech, is just a catch-all term that has come to mean *anything but indemnity*. But others contend that managing care, as an active term describing an active process, means integrating healthcare delivery and financing processes into one sophisticated design. Care integration and care process integration, they argue, are the hallmarks of productive managed care. True managed care goes way beyond discounting fee-for-service business or assembling a series of unlinked contracts or shifting risk onto unlinked, uncoordinated, unintegrated physicians and hospitals.

From a purely scientific perspective, managed care is an epidemiologic approach to deploying a group of healthcare services for a defined population. Economic benefits are reaped by managing care in clinically correct ways, not just by manipulating people and organizations to follow various misguided financial incentives.

Managed care must also be viewed as a largely regional marketplace phenomenon, at least for the time being. The practical definition of managed care varies markedly by region in the United States today. I am only half joking when I tell my colleagues how, whenever I hop on board an eastbound plane, I grow more and more brilliant as the flight approaches the Mississippi River. By the time we land in, say, Philadelphia, I'm convinced I'm the brightest managed-care mind anyone has ever laid eyes on. (More accurately, I am the one-eyed beggar in the land of the blind.)

East of the Mississippi River, any hastily organized (and usually unwelcome) attempt by payors to exert external influence on a physician's practice patterns, through such techniques as service preauthorization, in- and outpatient case management, peer review, profiling, and utilization management might be called managed care. In contrast, the conventional wisdom west of the Mississippi River, and most notably in my home state of California, is that dramatic changes in physician compensation (from fee-for-service to retrospective payment to prospective payment) are absolutely the keys to even more radical changes in physician practice patterns. These are changes we all need to achieve to meet the cost and quality imperatives of the present and future.

A Resolution

In the end, though, I cannot seriously entertain any definition of managed care that has been distilled to fit neatly into a single paragraph or that has been conceived from a lone perspective. That is why people write books, I suppose. For me, the only acceptable definition of managed care remains threefold as follows:

1. Select *higher principles* of managed care must inform our vision;
2. A handful of *basic techniques* must drive our daily operations; and
3. The shaping forces of the market must be fully understood and assimilated into our strategic thinking, if anyone expects to protect immediate business interests long enough to cultivate the higher principles and to fashion the basic techniques into useful tools.

The following discussion covers the higher principles and basic techniques of managed care. A broad variety of market forces are discussed in the remainder of this chapter and in Chapters 2 through 4; the discussion of market forces is then reprised in the final pages of the book, Chapter 9, and in the Afterword.

For the record, let this extensive coverage stand as my indivisible definition of managed care.

HIGHER PRINCIPLES

If the managed-care movement has a creed, it goes something like this:

We firmly believe that healthcare's greater good will best be served by delivering just the right healthcare, to just the right people, using just the right resources, in just the right settings, at the lowest possible costs.

Keeping this solemn vow means invoking certain higher principles that all payors, physicians, and providers can understand, incorporate into their daily lives and businesses, and return to periodically for inspiration.

I categorize the higher principles of managed care into the following five broad categories:

1. Prepayment, impanelment, and membership;
2. Managing health;
3. Defining and insuring populations;
4. Controlling risk; and
5. Processing information and managing outcomes.

Each of these five principles, you will notice, wages some new degree of control over healthcare processes and systems that now lack adequate control.

Prepayment, Impanelment, and Membership

Fundamental to the careful management of healthcare is a careful management of the finances and resources needed to serve a given population. In a sense, managed care is the purest imaginable arrangement between insurer and insured. It simplifies healthcare insurance by attaching a defined member population to a defined panel of providers and facilities. Members prepay a fixed premium per member per month, for which the managed-care organization—it may be a commercial or government payor, a physician group, a provider entity, or any combination of these—agrees to meet all of the membership population's healthcare needs through the eligible provider panel.

Payors' and providers' assumption of responsibility for a population's health in exchange for a fixed, prepaid "price per head" is often called *capitation*. And because the entire scheme is held together by any number of contracts between payors, providers, physicians, employers, and members, managed care is often, and perhaps most accurately, referred to as *contract healthcare*.

This changes everything we once knew about how to run a healthcare organization. Managed-care contracts and capitation are undermining the very notion of hospital service areas and market populations. We must now understand service populations defined not merely by geographic proximity, but by plan memberships and healthcare contracts.*

---

*Kurtenbach, Joan, and Trisha Warmoth, "Strategic planning futurists need to be capitation-specific and epidemiological," *Health Care Strategic Management*, 13:9, September 1995, p. 8.

Prepayment, impanelment, and membership must be accepted as the inviolable tenets of managed care practice. It astonishes me how often these principles have been bitterly challenged or relegated to a growing list of supposedly optional features. Prepaid capitated financing, a set panel of eligible providers, and a defined member population are three easy terms of contract healthcare that constitute a first corollary to managed care's humble creed.

Managing Health

Year by year we are discarding the time-honored "sickness" model of healthcare delivery and embracing a health management philosophy focused on preventing diseases and maintaining the health of defined populations. In the fee-for-service environment we built facilities and capabilities and hoped that people would need them. Managed care bets on health, not sickness. Soon we will not be planning for people to get sick; we will know what sicknesses people are likely to get and then plan to prevent or treat those ailments. The very moment an organization wholeheartedly accepts responsibility for the health of a population, its basic decision-making processes are transformed. This marks the beginning of the necessary transition from a sickness treatment to a health-management model.

Effective health management is a matter of common denominators. The basic technique is to slice the population into distinct risk groups such as age, sex, ethnicity, and disease. Then you must work to understand those clusters so you can tailor care delivery and reorganize to meet the needs of those populations. A few small risk groups account for the bulk of a membership's overall costs, and performing extremely well for these targeted subpopulations can do a world of good. This powerful concept often goes by the name *disease management.*

For a diabetic, for example, you can arrange a fine referral system that moves the patient seamlessly along a course of treatment. But you cannot really plot the right course until you have thought long and hard about the right way to care for the diabetic. There is your common denominator. Start thinking about variations in your clinical practice and in the design of your care support elements, such as X-rays, labs, and especially education and follow-up programs. Now we are really talking about integrating care and improving population health in discrete, manageable segments.

The actual mechanisms of everyday health management pose a considerable human challenge. If you reward physicians and other caregivers based on what happens to the health status of the populations for which they are responsible, then you have the right incentive system to move as far upstream in the disease process as you can. But managing health can only work when members themselves accept the risk for their own health and accept personal responsibility for prevention and early intervention. Then managed-care organizations will not be waiting forever for new injuries or illnesses to show up, they can start working ahead of the curve. Managed care's job is to keep the membership's health and well-being at the highest level possible, and sometimes one spirited educational campaign can do more than a thousand office visits or a thousand different drugs.

Managing health might soon mean exploring the psychosocial and even spiritual aspects of healthcare, too. A massage or aromatherapy session might offer a most effective course of prevention or primary care for some common ailments. Even a placebo effect can be a clinically and economically favorable effect.

The menu of alternative treatments goes deeper. Unihealth, for example, has been collecting data from some fascinating studies regarding the impact of prayer on health. Some 400 hospitalized post-heart attack patients in Florida were divided into two groups. One half were prayed for and the other half were not. The prayed-for group fared much better, experiencing significantly lower death rates and faster rates of recovery. Go figure. Ask doctors if they foresee a day when they will be writing prescriptions for visits to priests, rabbis, or counselors, and the heads start nodding. Together, patients and their spiritual or emotional guides can deal better with certain vital, extramedical aspects of health.

A fee-for-service system would never acknowledge the legitimacy of such extraclinical therapies. Minds start expanding in a true managed-care environment, where everyone is committed to finding the surest route to health and well-being. Someday we might see managed-care organizations partnering to tackle crime on the streets, drugs, lowering teenage pregnancy rates, getting kids to attend school, and other broader efforts designed to benefit community health. There can be more flexibility and more changes for the positive in a pure managed-care environment.

When I worked in Canada and the United Kingdom, the governments were busy setting incentives or disincentives that neatly circumnavigated the profit motive, although institutions and individuals could still make comfortable livings in healthcare. Until very recently though,

Canada and the United Kingdom had only succeeded at managing sickness, not health.

Canada was most fascinating. Ottawa decided how much it was willing to spend, then trimmed the budget to fit. But healthcare inflation rates marched up and up, the way they always had, because nothing whatsoever had changed at the end of the delivery line. The brightest opportunity lost came in the 1970s, when the system had performed better than the Gross Domestic Product rate of inflation, the benchmark we Yankees were using. The Canadians proceeded to beat their chests, instead of saying, "Okay, welcome to the plateau. Now what do we do for an encore?"

The United Kingdom is another story. You might call it a socialized version of the marketplace reform movement in the United States. When British citizens were absolutely fed up standing on long queues and getting shut out of the national healthcare system, they rose up and won fundamental reforms. A centralized National Health System, which was set up after the second World War as the government-run financing and budgeting arm, remained as the financing system. Pulling down a bureaucracy was no small task, but following the motto "the money will follow the patient" they began, as we have, to create fundamental changes in the responsiveness of providers, both physicians and hospitals, to better serve the population. They entered the era of managed financing about the same time we did. However, the reformers paid little or no regard to reforming the care delivery processes the government was financing. The British are trying, like we are trying, to paste new financing arrangements over old and persistent problems at the delivery system's root. Only now is the United Kingdom getting down to changing care delivery processes and, everyone hopes, moving toward managing the health of its population. If politics do not get in the way, the British have perhaps the best shot at creating managed care. They have the proper supply of primary care to specialist physicians and a proven ability to control capacity.

Managing health does pay; in fact, it pays quite handsomely. But it cannot offer the instant gratifications that too many demand. Can true managed-care health plans stick with the long view and still compete in a brisk market, where grabbing market share and lowering premiums seem so much more important? A health plan that intends to thrive in the managed-care business tomorrow has to maintain parts of its sickness system today. You cannot always manage population health, you must manage illness, too, and that is not managing care. But if one were to argue that the way a health plan stays in business is to provide no care to the healthy and no care to the chronically ill, pretty soon all those chronic cases would fit your acutely ill-risk profile. It is not a viable competitive approach. Plans will not survive in tomorrow's marketplace if they refuse preventive services to a healthy population that wants to stay that way.

True managed-care organizations are pushing to manage not only costs but quality and outcomes. Managing care implies managing the care outcomes, managing health for a population that has entrusted its health-care to your organization. It is not about avoiding risk or limiting services or resources. How do we prevent people from coming in to use services? How do we keep people healthier? How do we manage the population to achieve these goals? If we spend 50% of our costs on, say, just 6% of our enrollment, how can we do a better job of managing the select diseases, such as diabetes, asthma, HIV, AIDS, and chronic conditions that afflict those 6%?

Obstetrics is a notably high-cost item. For such a standard procedure, delivering a baby consumes a surprising lot of resources. The managed-care community has gotten past all the controversy over the mandatory 48-hour lengths of stay. We are going to do what is right for the member, most plans concur. We do not push people out if they are not ready. But we must find ways of better managing obstetric health. We need the right information, properly sorted. How do costs break down by diagnosis and by physician? We can use the answers as an educational tool to better train our physicians regarding what they can do differently based on the performance of their peers. Time and time again the seasoned health plan executive has learned a basic lesson: create a positive incentive, based on sound clinical science, and physicians will respond.

Enlightened plans also know that the primary care gatekeeper model, characteristic of managed-care lite and medium marketplaces, is seriously flawed. The whole gatekeeping structure was erected to block access to specialists, solely to save money. It should be intuitively obvious that, through constant repetition, one gets very good at doing specialized procedures. Early managed care efforts have been asking primary-care specialists to do more subspecialty work than they are probably comfortable handling. Quality of care has probably suffered, though you hear different stories all around. In the literature, you often hear that gatekeeper models achieve higher quality, patient satisfaction, and lower hospital utilization. Credit should not go to gatekeeping but to the rigorous assignment of each patient to a personal physician, which instantly improves care and access. Improved outcomes beyond primary care are but an indirect result of gatekeeping.

In a more enlightened approach, the patient can still choose a specialist, perhaps with the aid of her or his primary-care physician but without so many hurdles to access. Such enlightenment might come with the next generation of managed-care techniques, featuring specialist capitation. We can re-incentivize specialists. Under a fee-for-service scheme, specialists are motivated to treat patients in order to *get* revenue; under a prepaid, capitated scheme, specialists would be motivated to treat patients most appropriately in order to *keep* revenue.

Defining and Insuring Populations

A new actuarial and epidemiological science is born with the definition of the covered population enrolled in a prepaid health product. A more strictly held patient population lends itself to closer study, with more definitive results, so providers can weigh their risks in more quantifiable terms. Coupled with the classic service population characteristics, demographics, socioeconomics, and geographic distribution, traditionally studied in healthcare market research, such epidemiologic data will become instrumental in managing key areas of clinical and business risk. Epidemiologic information needs to be updated, tested, and monitored periodically to ensure that it is current, to monitor factors that may be causing changes in the market, and to measure your progress against key indicators.*

The right system collects all the appropriate data, data not only on populations but also data that will tell you how to deal with individual patients. Only with such a rich store of population- and member-specific data can a managed-care organization establish best practices, watch for variability, communicate, and continuously improve. Reliable comparative data is tough to gather in a fee-for-service environment. You also need utilization review data that is perceived as more friend than foe.

Insurance is not the endpoint. Insurance is a mechanism that allows you to provide the appropriate care, in the appropriate place, in the most cost-effective and efficient way. And so the intent is not to think about creating a wide range of insurance products but, rather, to ensure that the financing systems you have in place do indeed enable you to deliver the very best care to the population.

Insurance actuaries use mathematical probability to project the financial effects that various events, such as birth, marriage, sickness,

---

*Kurtenbach, p. 9.

accident, fire, liability, retirement, and death have on insurance, benefit plans, and other financial security systems. Actuaries examine a population's history then draw a straight line toward the inevitable future.

Epidemiologists, on the other hand, examine a population's history then figure out how to divert that line toward an alternative, healthier future. Epidemiology promises to be a much more powerful tool than marketing. And there is a lot of money to be made by predicting the incidence and prevalence of certain troublesome diseases and conditions, when confidently organizing your service offerings to handle that expected use.

An epidemiologist seeks out the root causes of avoidable healthcare costs. If factory employees suffer a lot of back problems, for instance, an astute health plan epidemiologist can visit the assembly line and work with the employer to reduce the risk of back injury. If neonatal intensive care utilization seems too high, the astute plan can work with obstetricians to do everything medically appropriate to keep infants *in utero*. Given both the high risk of premature deliveries and the astronomical cost of a single day in the neonatal intensive care unit, such efforts pay big human and economic dividends.

Having worked and lived eleven years in Canada and three years in the United Kingdom, I observed that epidemiologists were regarded as important physicians in those societies. Here in the United States, I cannot recall meeting anybody so bold as to stand up and announce, "I am an epidemiologist." I am sure they exist, but apparently they are not attending the high-level planning meetings I do. Things must change. We must begin studying our subscriber demographics in earnest, breaking populations down into categories, such as geography, employer, and disease state that make the most sense to those responsible for managing health.

To manage health, you need to gather two sets of information: (1) population characteristics and (2) provider performance. Depending on how large the population is, look at differences among geographies, cultures, and industries. Look for reasons behind any differences in the way people use care or get care. To measure provider performance, one can rely on standard productivity measures. But apply such methods retrospectively rather than as rigid rules. All the latest profiles and quantitative methods are just marvelous for looking at things collectively. But when the figures look wrong, do not try to fix the figures. Go behind the numbers. It could be you are not counting right or you did not define things right. Remember that behaviors drive the figures, not vice versa. We should be managing care, not numbers.

In the final analysis, managing health means protecting the best interests of the subscriber. Wherever the subscriber's interests conflict with others' interests, carefully examine the roots of the conflict. Conflicts with employers? Employers want their employees to be happy. Conflicts with physicians and providers? Doctors want to make their patients healthy. A strong health plan plants a financial umbrella under which such potential conflicts are displaced by closely aligned motives and missions.

Controlling Risk

In a way, all of us in the healthcare industry are just now learning the classic business techniques and positive attitudes that so many others, especially manufacturers, have long used to stay viable in their markets and industries. Take Motorola. Their first cellular phone took two weeks to build. Through the innovations of Continuous Quality Improvement and other proven business techniques, their latest model takes just two hours to make, and it is cheaper and more reliable.

In healthcare, too, both nonprofits and for-profits are achieving continuous quality improvements and higher productivity, which have yielded lower overall costs and lower labor costs as a percentage of revenue, a figure that has fallen every year for the last five years. And everyone knows they have got to perform even better next year. In large part, these recent quality and productivity improvements in healthcare stem from the improved control of business risks.

There are ethical and unethical ways of controlling business risk. It is unethical to control business risk simply by controlling the risk pool. That kind of skating and slicing is an insurance approach to risk. Another unethical control method is economic credentialing, in which you gather data on the expenses of all the providers in your system, then periodically eliminate the most expensive culprits. That is cheating.

The true managed-care model controls business risk by improving quality, constantly narrowing its variations in clinical practice, driving always toward what is most acceptable and appropriate given the current state of understanding about how to manage a certain disease. Eliminating the troublesome variations that are not grounded in medical science, through professional dialogue and protocol development, is the surest way to cut costs and reduce risk. Less variation in clinical practices also reduces variations in care-support systems, including diagnostic and treatment services, appointment systems, education support, and such.

Outcomes research also informs the preventive and clinical practice, narrowing variation yet further.

As physician groups download risk through capitated prepayment, which after all is the real thrust of good managed care, they must understand precisely what they are getting into. You cannot dabble in capitation. Successfully taking on risk means learning a whole new set of skills, especially the actuarial skills to calculate Incurred But Not Reported (IBNR) claims.

Most physician groups think IBNR is a railroad! In truth, IBNR measures the gap between the prepayment and the actual receipt of a claim for an encounter. If a group does not have a handle on its IBNR accounts, its financial picture may look too rosy. Balancing debits and credits is trickier under a prepaid arrangement, and expert money management is all the more important.

A physician group serving a larger population enjoys less fluctuation in business risk. Operating on a broader scale, the group is less susceptible to the dramatic impact of large cases. When they do face a large case, some groups have been successful in negotiating favorable contracts or special rates. In negotiating a global fee for a transplant, for example, one fee covers physician care for the whole case, even if the patient has to come back for another transplant.

Customer satisfaction is another key to controlling business risk. Keeping a customer is always better than losing one and having to win a new one. And customer satisfaction takes a lot more than wearing a smiley-face button. You have to build and tend a disciplined process for measuring, tracking, and constantly improving satisfaction.

If you operate multiple sites, branding is an invaluable technique to manage customer satisfaction. Like a fast-food diner who knows the burger he picks up at a drive-thru across the street tastes the same as one served over the counter at the same franchise across town, a patient who visits Medical Group A one morning should enjoy a comfortably similar experience when she visits Clinic B later that afternoon. Affiliated facilities should look and feel about the same to the people who staff them and use them.

When I used to take foreign visitors on tours of different FHP clinics, now Talbert Clinics, I was struck by the homogenous culture they had established. The personnel all dressed the same, the clerks even looked the same, and the facilities surely were identical in color and decor. They could plop a preplanned, prefabricated facility down anywhere, with the standard three examining rooms per physician and not a worry about un-proven designs. Every detail, from documents to architecture, is repli-cated. All exam rooms are identical, so when a doctor fills in at another facility he knows right where to reach for a tongue depressor. He can spring into action without missing a beat.

Branding has its hazards, too. Consider the Mayo Clinic's experi-ence in Jacksonville and Phoenix. Many would give Mayo pride of place on the short list of America's finest healthcare institutions. But they had difficulty transplanting their culture outside Minnesota. Beyond a core of Mayo-trained physicians, the facilities soon found trouble drawing from the unfamiliar social environments of Jacksonville and Phoenix, they lit-tle understood the cultural differences.

When you are starting a new organization, you enjoy design opportu-nities you can never replicate later on. The Japanese auto companies seem to understand this principle. When they moved into Tennessee, the govern-ment gave them all sorts of flack for so painstakingly testing and selecting their United States employees. Just hire our people and run your factories, the government complained. No, said the Japanese. We are here to live, and we are here to make the best cars. So they took the heat, toiled away at trans-planting their corporate culture, and have proven quite successful.

As part of the effort to dovetail cultures and control risk, internal audit functions need to be beefed up. It is not so much a tighter policing that is needed but, again, that common look, feel, and function. When you are prepaid, smarter routine audit practices can squeeze out an extra per-centage point or two in annual interest, a fairly significant amount of bonus income for some providers.

One health plan went so far as market testing how long it could hold back its per diem payments before hospitals screamed. Starting at both ends of the spectrum, 60 days and 20 days, they simply ratcheted inward a day at a time, finally arriving at the ideal cycle of 32 days. So now the plan pays every hospital bill when it is exactly 32 days old, and everyone is happy. That is managing risk the easy way! You do not want to hurt your partners, but you do want to manage your money wisely. Providers had better learn the same lesson. Perhaps you need to pay your specialists in 28 days, or risk losing them. How will you ever know unless you test the waters?

Thanks to this wonderful Information Age of ours, and in particular the radical improvement lately in managed-care information systems, we enjoy the unprecedented opportunity to examine cost by CPT code, by

ICD-9-DM code, by provider, and by specialty. It is a much less complex task to identify the financial risk. Once you quantify it, you must work to sensitize physicians to manage it. Physicians are the key. Now, if only we could get patients to manage financial risk from the source, that would be a neat trick!

Processing Information and Managing Outcomes

The outcomes management revolution is being fueled by a rich new lode of highly meaningful information. So far the industry has focused exclusively on the industrial engineering solution, that is retooling processes to establish higher standards for superior efficiency. New information will inspire us to think outside that old box and pursue a broader vision. Over the next few years, advanced managed-care organizations will be investing in electronic, member-based medical records linked to protocol databases. We will have all the vital information on hand and be able to measure it and profile it against what actually happens. It is going to be phenomenal to truly manage outcomes by creating claims histories, data warehouses, and comparison tools with ready access to our full continuum of costs and protocols. And by keeping electronic member health records for an entire community with, say, two million lives, you will really have a strong basis for statistically meaningful comparison. Then you can institute an education process that drives the information home to physicians and incorporates their feedback regarding variations. The variations in clinical practice are sometimes wild, and until now there has been no convincing incentive for physicians to change that. Solid clinical information on large populations will have a very positive effect on both the cost and the quality sides of the equation. And once we can track outcomes from the beginning of the care process to the middle to the end, the process will be ripe for the kinds of constant improvement we have all wished for.

Managed care is really all about measuring health status and managing outcomes. Constantly test physician care against the best demonstrated practices, as you currently understand them. Develop a better and better understanding of outcomes given population size and, as you develop the proper metrics, feature that information in how you gauge the very success of your organization. Health Plan Employer Data and Information Set (HEDIS) measures care processes more than it does health status, precisely, but process measures are rather directly linked to health status.

We might as well begin this managed-care education at the educational source. Today our medical academies serve the interests of individuals who live mainly to do clinical research. A proper managed-care technique will put the research horse back in front of the cart. The research effort should rightly begin with a close study of the academy's faculty practice plan's membership, proceed to identify specific problems among that population, then send researchers on the quest for the most practical, medically sound, and economically responsible solutions. To fund such population- and outcomes-focused research, some propose a premium "tax" that earmarks monies for targeted research activities. Essentially, the membership would fund the research of its own health problems, as well as basic medical research. The managed-care organization would oversee the allocation of funds and monitor progress. And if the managed-care academics play it smart, they could raise more funds by taxing premiums than they do in today's grant system. Researchers would be required to report periodically to a group of peers and plan representatives, who will challenge the utility of the research.

Some hope that outcomes data will help consumers pick a health plan. Plans routinely keep track of customer satisfaction data, like complaints and waiting times, but these are hardly measures of good health. Health Maintenance Organizations (HMOs) provide an organizational arrangement in which we can measure, epidemiologically, the quality of care they provide to large populations. We have lacked quality control because we have lacked the computing power to study populations and perform meaningful comparisons to meaningful benchmark data. Patients have never had objective quality comparisons that talk about results. Your average consumer is going to be surprised and confused when they get hold of the easily readable information, revealing just how much uncertainty there is in medical care and how many tradeoffs clinicians make every day. Suddenly people will gain a frightening insight into what medical professionals do, why they do it, and the real chances of success or failure.*

We are on the cusp of having much better data. We are only a couple of years away from truly valid outcomes data. We would all love reliable cost data across the full continuum of care, but that revolution is in the development stage. Better physician profiling information is another dream within reach.

---

*Paul Ellwood, MD, "Commentary: The father of the HMO mulls quality measures," *Modern Healthcare*, 22 April 1996, p. 33.

Managing health means managing outcomes. Very few have the resources to do it. Outcomes measurement must be coordinated with practice guideline development. If you have not established a guideline and measured compliance with that guideline, and then worked to win better compliance, you do not know what is driving your outcome, even if you measure it. Managing health has to happen. If we do not do it, but continue to focus on costs alone, then our ultimate outcome is bound to be failure.

Two sports analogies spring to mind, if you will indulge me. The first analogy we shall name "The Fallacy of the First-down Marker." On a close call for the first down, football referees usher in the Bureau of Standards and Measures for a laser-precise verdict. After a grueling battle over nearly ten yards of muddy turf, a fraction of an inch counts. I am telling you, the umpire has no clothes! No one dares mention the gross imprecisions involved at every step in this time-honored system of measures. Finding the ball under a pileup, spotting it accurately on the field, walking the sacred chains and scepters from the sidelines to the scene, the whole ritual welcomes significant margins of error, right up until the time arrives to determine the final outcome. One minute the official is pacing off a penalty, "exactly" half the distance to the goal line, and the next minute he is holding up thumb and forefinger to indicate third down and angstroms to go.

What good will all the sophisticated analytical tools and outcomes data in the world do us if we do not also have reliable base data, describing members' original health status, and routine clinical protocols, establishing the core processes by which members' health is restored.

The second analogy we shall name "Spot Bowling for Dollars." Bowlers are of two breeds. Pin bowlers aim the ball at a pocket among the set pins, way down at the end of the alley. Spot bowlers aim the ball across the arrows painted just a few feet from the foul line. Assuming one can rely on a consistent grip, approach, stroke, and release (like the "repeating swing" every golfer works so hard to cultivate) frame after frame any bowler will find it much easier to hit the closer mark. The score may still be counted at the pins (where Newton's Laws forever reign) and the reward money counted in dollars, but success is measured by the contestant's ability to hit consistently within a sliver to the right or left of the arrow.

Here, then, is a fitting corollary to Andrew Carnegie's brilliant maxim: Mind your costs and the profits will take care of themselves. In managed care, too, costs demand constant monitoring. But you can turn an even tidier profit by making health, not costs or profits, the primary goal. But we must be of two conscientious minds when it comes to playing such a high-stakes game, where outcomes mean not only dollars but lives. Mind your quality of care, we add, and your clinical and economic outcomes will take care of themselves.

Managed-care information systems today are all based on claims processing. We are not yet able to integrate claims or encounter data with satisfaction, outcomes, or hospital data. Until all these databases are brought together into a relational database, providers are not going to have the right information at their disposal, that is, the information we need to truly manage health. The cavalry, riding to our rescue through all this dust, may be a Microsoft or an Oracle.

BASIC TECHNIQUES

Once an organization has embraced managed care in the purity of its concept, or at least come to terms with the changing reality, the more difficult struggle begins. New ways of thinking demand new ways of doing business and delivering healthcare.

I count, at least, the following eight distinct tools that every managed-care organization must soon acquire and eventually master:

1. Education, screening, and prevention;
2. Case management;
3. Utilization review and management;
4. Clinical pathways;
5. Continuous quality improvement;
6. Organizational change management;
7. Incentive systems; and
8. Population study and epidemiologic analysis.

Each of these basic techniques, you might have deduced, supports one or more of managed care's higher principles.

Education, Screening, and Prevention

Managed care makes its biggest impact on the healthy population and the subpopulations at risk for certain troublesome diseases and conditions.

The keys to preserving health are prevention, early detection, and self-management. Achieving these objectives will require a whole new attitude toward member education and support. People must be informed, motivated, and trained to become active members of the care team. Most will be glad to know their own risks, prevent illness, stop chronic disease from progressing, and self-rehabilitate whenever possible.

Implementing effective education, screening, and prevention campaigns ranks among managed care's greatest challenges. So many other matters seem more pressing in healthcare today. Ounces of prevention and pounds of cure do not figure in healthcare's new metric system. Actually changing the behaviors of vast populations will require the concerted efforts of payors, providers, and physicians as well as the creative use of every medium that might best relay our crucial health messages.

Case Management

Good case management is part and parcel of good managed care. After all, healthcare is really only manageable one case at a time, case after case after case.

A case manager may be deployed by the payor, provider, or physician to guide the member through the most appropriate course of interventions and referrals. Case management thus puts a human face on managed healthcare. Yes, patients today need a trusted guide in their journey from one discipline to another and from site to site in an ever-expanding continuum of care. More to the point, case management supplies the indispensable means by which clinical guidelines can be operationalized and care delivery can be coordinated and optimized to produce superior outcomes.

Although case management is our best weapon against a fragmented healthcare system, it serves the interests of consumers rather than the needs of the system. Along with the consumer advocate, ombudsperson, clinical and system expert, the case manager is a welcome hand in the managed-care arena.

Utilization Review and Management

Managed care reaps significant savings by monitoring the utilization of resources and enforcing adherence to stricter protocols that improve quality by reducing process variations. In fee-for-service systems, doctors consider utilization review a police force. Under capitation, where everyone's at risk, utilization review serves the mutual interests of payors, providers, and physicians. It can really work when everyone pitches in.

But even the most advanced organizations are not profiling performance very well, giving doctors useful, actionable information on how they are performing compared to their colleagues in terms of patient satisfaction, clinical outcomes, compliance with practice guidelines, utilization of resources, and overall cost of care. Profiling should be done every month and, in a managed-care heavy environment, physician performance and behavior should gain our undivided attention. Doctors should be reviewing the data and producing reports on their peers, such as internists on internists, pediatricians on pediatricians, and cardiologists on cardiologists.

Furthermore, managed care expands the traditional purview of utilization management. We must begin to look beyond standards of diagnosis, treatment, and therapy to incorporate the measurable outcomes of preventive and rehabilitative courses. Physicians need to learn what works best and earliest in the life-cycle of a given ailment.

Clinical Pathways

Better understanding the health needs of a member population can have a wonderfully clarifying effect on clinical practice. Physicians today are embracing new means of coordinating care for superior quality, efficiency, and cost-effectiveness. Clinical pathways, care protocols, physician guidelines, call them what you will, are a few standard operating procedures that can do a world of good for the quality of care and the preservation of health.

Clinical pathways also constitute the managed-care physician's major contribution to payor and provider strategies. Pathways are the means by which payors and providers can plan how best to absorb the community's predicted demand for specific healthcare services. Whatever the demand, a well-thought-out clinical pathway will make it possible to accurately measure outcomes and achieve maximum efficiencies and improvements. A sound plan manifests itself in sound clinical pathways. And sound pathways are driven by physicians and constantly informed by fresh clinical and economic outcomes data.

Again, the advent of wholly integrated delivery systems will facilitate an expansion of pathways, as physicians can follow members from health to risk, to primary care, to acute care, to rehabilitation and, ultimately, a return to health. Pathways worth following will be blazed across integrated networks, without discrimination as to payor, setting, or caregiver.

Continuous Quality Improvement

By now the principles of Continuous Quality Improvement (CQI) are a time-honored concept in American business, even in the healthcare industry. Next, mere principles must be honed into everyday tools and techniques. Process tune-ups and quality improvements mean nothing if they cannot be linked to the right measured outcomes, namely lower costs and improved health. The information systems and management innovations we need to do the CQI job right might be years in the designing.

Organizational Change Management

The proliferation of capitated, prepaid healthcare financing should urge providers to get to know their populations' changing needs and their own organizations' flexibility to constantly adapt to serve those changing needs. A health-managing organization looks outward then inward. The more thorough its epidemiologic and demographic studies, the better its chances of assembling just the right resources, just in time. In an era when every investment in facilities, technologies, and human resources must be scrutinized in light of precisely calibrated budgets and strategies, one's intelligence and confidence must be high.

After clairvoyant prediction and crafty planning comes expert management. Building and running a more sophisticated network whose resources will be constantly shifting toward preventive care, wellness, home, rehabilitative, and self-care will require brand new skills and, perhaps, brand-new managers.

Chapter 8 more fully explores the vital discipline of organizational change management in the emerging managed-care environment.

Incentives

Monetary and professional incentives (and disincentives) loom large in popular impressions of and approaches to managed care today. With the new emphasis on prevention, early detection, and intervention, such ill-wrought incentive structures are straining to the breaking point. True managed care imposes only positive reinforcements of practices and behaviors that improve health.

Next, incentive structures will reach out to healthy, acute, and chronic populations and their provider institutions. We are spreading the risk for health across the system, and individual and group risks can be quantified and translated into newly shared responsibilities for effective prevention and intervention.

Population Study and Epidemiologic Analysis

We are entering a Renaissance of public health. Just as actuaries have long studied the insurance risks of general populations, epidemiologists today can study the future health risks of a defined member population. Then they can work with managed-care planners to segment the overall population into specific risk categories, predict the demand for certain healthcare services, outline the likeliest episodes of care, plan the most effective preventions and interventions, and prepare the organization to assemble the right resources at the right time.

More powerful, faster information processing capabilities promise to make epidemiologic science an uncannily accurate and useful tool. In classifying population segments according to risk, we will see the most fundamental change in the way we view the management of health. Once a managed-care organization familiarizes itself with its high-risk populations and individuals, it can begin to monitor the success of current practices and then refine them or tailor new practices that improve health.

S U M M A R Y

Managed care's prescription for thoughtful prevention and superior efficiency offers the most prudent remedy, both clinically and economically, for contemporary healthcare's serious woes. But just how novel is this supposedly young science and business? Speaking quite literally, do we not already manage care, and have we not always done so?

Yes we do and, yes, we always have. The thinkers and laborers of human medicine have managed care for as long as there has been some kind of healthcare needing some kind of management. Tribal shamans, medieval barbers, battlefield nurses, country doctors, hospital-nursing unit clerks, case workers, and integrated delivery systems, haven't they all, in their own fashion, carefully managed the care they provided? And managed care proper, in the guise of prepaid public health plans, has been kicking around since World War II. So there must be more to today's managed-care revolution than can neatly be contained in two words lifted from the hardest-working of vocabularies.

What is so remarkably different about managing healthcare today is the confluence of a few newfound shortcomings in our healthcare system and a few brand-new capabilities to address those issues. Both our need and our ability to manage care stand at an all-time high. Specifically, the present healthcare environment is characterized as follows:

- A changing economic reality in which all purchasers of healthcare, such as insurers, employers, and consumers insist on superior value;
- The bold new promise that we can ascertain, in the richest imaginable detail and on a statistically meaningful scale, the actual health risks and needs of entire communities;
- A refreshingly aggressive new stance on public health, epitomized by an ever stronger emphasis on education, screening, and prevention; and
- The advent of powerful information technologies and analytical techniques, enabling health organizations to interpret population health data, quickly retool and reorganize to best address specific risks and needs, and ultimately, act decisively to preserve health.

Managed care's restless quest for value has become an especially pressing necessity in light of our rapidly aging population and alarming demographic shifts. Simply put, more and more people are going to need healthcare in the years ahead, yet more and more will find themselves unable to finance adequate healthcare coverage via personal resources, traditional employee insurance benefits, or government social endowments.

The future practice of managed care will be the net yield of these marketplace realities and other shaping forces at work today. By enthusiastically adopting the higher principles and creatively applying the basic techniques we have explored in this chapter, we are preparing the way for a lasting change whose ultimate beneficiaries will be the next generation of American healthcare consumers. Tomorrow's industry pioneers will traverse a landscape made truly hospitable for truly managed care.

2

CHAPTER

Forces at Work Today

At this late date, the first meaningful reports are just now arriving from the managed-care frontier, and the news ranges from excellent to mixed. A few advanced regional markets have demonstrated managed care's astounding potential to cut costs while improving health. But for every rousing success, it seems, there has been a dear price to pay, a new hurdle to surmount; for every noble principle and effective technique there has appeared some misrepresentative abuser or outspoken critic; for every new clinical or business conception there has arisen a serious misperception in the industry, in the media, or in the public mind.

Indeed, these are exciting but confusing times in American healthcare. Getting at the hardest kernels of truth about managed care, as an integral social, business, and political phenomenon of our national future, will require our deeper understanding of the powerful forces at work in today's regional and local healthcare marketplaces.

Chief among these shaping forces is the imminent extinction of what we used to call the hospital. A sprawling variety of more attractive alternative care settings, as well as innovative ownership and control arrangements, have profoundly altered the way we must think about how, why, and where we deliver healthcare services in the next century. Specifically, our entire healthcare community must adapt to the following three pre-vailing trends in the provider sector:

1. Hospitals, through integration and the incessant shifting of traditional acute care into alternative settings, are fast becoming "centers of health" rather than sickness care facilities;
2. Acute care institutions are downsizing constantly and becoming more expense-intensive care units; and
3. Vacated acute care spaces are being filled by ambulatory care, skilled nursing, extended care, and health diagnostic centers.

This ongoing dissolution of our classic healthcare-provider institutions is sending shockwaves across the entire industry and throughout our society.

In this chapter we ponder the relevant economic, social, market, op-erating, and regulatory issues that are shaping the managed-care land-scape. Of special interest is how providers, payors, and physicians, in un-precedented and often troublesome collaboration, are answering these powerful trends with powerful new strategies.

MANAGED CARE BY THE NUMBERS

Member enrollment in Health Maintenance Organizations (HMOs) has steadily and dramatically increased since 1976, as shown in Table 2–1. HMOs currently cover more than 50 million lives, representing nearly 70% of all working Americans. We can rather confidently predict that HMOs will cover some 100 million American lives by the turn of the century. And the bigger managed-care picture is just as bright. Currently HMOs represent 29% of all health-plan enrollees, with managed care "hybrids," such as preferred provider organizations, representing another 40%.

This mass migration toward managed care, though certainly quite impressive, can be misleading. So much of the managed-care arena re-mains almost completely unexplored, and a strong backlash might make it difficult to keep spreading the good word. Yes, the success of managed care companies appears to stem directly from their ability to control healthcare costs, which had escalated so alarmingly in the 1980s under traditional indemnity coverage. But true managed care is not all about costs. Studies are beginning to show lower mortality rates in advanced managed-care markets, even as inpatient costs per member and hospital stays decrease. Moreover, plan members themselves have consistently

TABLE 2-1

Growth in HMO Enrollment, 1976-1995

	HMO Enrollees (in millions)		HMO Enrollees (in millions)
1976	6.0	1986	25.7
1977	6.3	1987	29.3
1978	7.5	1988	32.7
1979	8.2	1989	34.7
1980	9.1	1990	36.5
1981	10.2	1991	38.6
1982	10.8	1992	41.4
1983	12.5	1993	45.2
1984	15.1	1994	51.1
1985	18.9	1995	56.0

Sources:

Health Affairs, Summer 1988, for years ending 30 June 1976-1987.

GHAA's National Directory of HMOs database, for years ending 31 December 1988-1994. (Note: The GHAA, or Group Health Association of America, has since become the American Association of Health Plans.)

Estimate based on *GHAA's 1994 HMO Performance Report,* for the year ending 1 October 1995.

expressed a positive experience with managed care and a general satisfaction with service and coverage.

ECONOMIC AND SOCIAL ISSUES

On the national stage, healthcare plays a leading role in the overall economy and in our basic social workings. The managed-care movement cannot help but also be a significant economic and social movement. At least the following two truths seem incontrovertible in this regard:

- Most investments in healthcare quality pay big dividends, both economic and social; and
- Excellent healthcare does little good if it cannot also be made widely accessible and easily affordable.

High expectations for quality, accessibility, and affordability have colored the managed-care debate from the very beginning and will be perennial issues for the industry to tackle.

Cost versus Quality?

Cost concerns are taking a back seat to quality issues in healthcare today. Customers in the growing managed-care market, who once focused almost exclusively on cost containment as the criterion for selecting one insurer over another, now do their level best to make selections based primarily on a demonstrated high quality of service. Employers have come to realize that employee productivity relates directly to employee health, and better healthcare may be a most powerful productivity enhancer. Especially as premiums have relatively leveled off in the past two years, customers (specifically employers) are now beginning to focus more on quality. As competition for membership intensifies, the likeliest winners will be insurers that can consistently provide the highest quality of service at the best level of value.

Balancing purchasers' expectations with investors' focus on profits, costs, and revenue growth will be a main challenge for the industry in the years to come. Over the next several years, as information on quality becomes publicly available, consumers at long last may gain access to the information they need to select a plan based on their own good judgment. Payors may need to reshuffle their priorities rapidly to succeed under this new public scrutiny.

Yet costs will continue to trouble the managed-care movement. Many HMOs have found it more difficult than anticipated to curtail unnecessary and unnecessarily costly hospitalizations, treatments, procedures, therapies, and prescriptions. In times of heated competition to build membership, health plans had little choice but to take the hit with small or no rate hikes. Now they face an ever mounting pressure to raise rates, as profit margins and stock prices decline.

Drug costs remain perhaps the most vexing issue for most health plans. Even though they represent an extremely small proportion of total health costs, drug prescriptions are among the hardest elements to control. HMOs continue to enjoy success in persuading hospitals and doctors to hand over deep fee discounts, but drug companies have proven to be shrewd negotiators. The major pharmaceutical houses, which once gladly cut prices for HMOs in the hope of getting more business from their members, are driving tougher bargains and demanding firm guarantees of brisker sales. Some HMOs cannot or will not provide such assurances.*

---

*Associated Press, online newswire story, New York, 3 October 1996, by Steve Sakson.

We are emerging from a prolonged "crunching down" period, in which there has actually been a surprising decline in premiums. But now, if the market starts to loosen up a bit, will indemnity plan and Preferred Provider Organizations (PPO) rates start to rise faster than the HMO premiums? If the gap grows wide enough, price alone will drive the population into membership and drive the hybrid carriers into true managed care. Finally, we could start penetrating managed care's virgin market, those 35% or so who have not tried an HMO yet. Judging by the California experience, once the cost shakeout is over, and premiums have fallen down around $100 per member per month, a market stabilizes. Purchasers are then driven much more by marketing and quality than purely by cost.

In spirit, at least, managed care amounts to the healthcare industry selectively emulating the best practices of the manufacturing industry. Manufacturers today are constantly working to figure out how they can make a better product at a lower cost. In healthcare this struggle really means declaring freedom from the specific mechanisms of delivery and knowing that, as the science improves and as our understanding of resource utilization improves, we can find more efficient ways of delivering the same or better quality care.

Improved clinical quality and lower costs are by no means mutually exclusive propositions. The fact is, the surest, most responsible way to lower the cost of healthcare is to improve the effectiveness, efficiency, and outcomes of care processes.

Accessibility and Affordability

Universal access to healthcare has been a hot topic for many years, and the issue achieved an even higher profile when universal healthcare became a major feature of President Clinton Administration's national healthcare reform package.

Recent trends in corporate downsizing, layoffs, outplacement, self-employment, and outright unemployment have made access to healthcare a major issue for many people. Healthcare insurance becomes a new worry when it is no longer a benefit of employment but, rather, a policy to be secured on the open market. In the course of the recent debate over reform, insurers' traditional means of underwriting, particularly the exclusion of coverage for preexisting conditions and specific diseases, have become socially unacceptable. Also, the increasing mobility of employees in an uncertain employment environment has made portability and noncancellation important and popular features to many consumers.

It is very likely these forces will completely transform the product design, pricing, and underwriting of group and individual health plans through the turn of the century. More important, employees' and nonemployees' widespread concerns about coverage has built up the pressure on states and the federal government to participate in creating new solutions.

MARKET ISSUES

As a marketplace phenomenon, managed care has become a force to be reckoned with on a number of fronts, including the following:

- Mergers, acquisitions, and joint ventures;
- Integrated delivery systems;
- Provider-based HMOs;
- Medicare privatization;
- 24-hour coverage;
- Image, reputation, and financial strength; and
- Globalization and international ventures.

Our discussion of managed care's chief market issues may be fit conveniently, if not quite so neatly, into these broad categories.

Accelerating Mergers, Acquisitions, and Joint Ventures

Mergers and acquisitions of hospitals, physician groups, and laboratories have become commonplace. Everyone should have seen it coming. Such a vast industry, consuming about one-seventh of our national output, simply could not go on any longer operating as a collection of tiny, inefficient enterprises.

Many insurers and managed care companies, in a quest to broaden their geographic or demographic reach in the market, are turning to mergers and acquisitions. Joining forces is often seen as a way of expanding marketing capabilities while simultaneously providing an opportunity to achieve improved economies of scale. Usually, a strong expertise in a specific market niche, or a concentration that is complementary to the acquiring firm's book of business, provides rationale enough for the deal.

Significant mergers and acquisitions between insurance companies and managed-care companies have been the recent trend. Insurance mergers have been linked with, and appear to be a result of, the rapid consolidation among hospitals, doctors, and medical suppliers. Additionally, insurance companies offer attractive benefits coverage in other lines, including wealth accumulation and savings, death protection, and disability. Insurers view strategic partnerships with niche managed-care companies as a way to provide "one-stop" access to customers and to feed their seemingly insatiable desire to gain access to HMO markets already tapped by the managed-care companies.

Proponents believe that, although cultural gaps will be a challenge to overcome, consumers will benefit from cost savings, expertly run HMO operations, and quality of care; the merged entities believe profits will come from cost savings, economies of scale, and cross-selling of other products. Opponents worry that consumer choice may eventually be reduced to managed-care products (indemnity products will become obsolete) and providers and employers alike may be left without bargaining power. Regardless, it is clear that merging aggressively-managed HMO companies with highly capitalized and surplus-rich insurance companies promises to be a constant challenge for the merging entities. They must figure out how to apply the effective medical management capabilities of HMO companies to often less tightly run indemnity insurers' networks, while maintaining the typically low medical loss ratios associated with the acquired managed-care companies.

The Rise of the Integrated Delivery System

It is wonderful that the healthcare market has found so many different ways of financing, insuring, and contracting. But that is not managing care. Integrating the healthcare delivery system is the way you manage care. And no amount of merging, acquiring, and joint venturing can create a truly integrated managed care environment.

Integrated delivery represents an even greater promise for managing care to lower costs and improve quality. In fact, managed care *is* integration; you cannot have one without the other. An integrated delivery system allows the plan member to proceed from picking up the phone, to describing a symptom, to getting the definitive care, to enjoying the best possible outcome. All the elements along this seamless roadway to health must be wholly integrated.

But for all the talk lately about integrated delivery systems, they simply do not exist. Yet. It is one thing to achieve integration for a small population, in a single physician practice, for instance. It is quite another to do it across a population of two or six million.

The more we talk about managing the health of vast populations, the more we should be talking about targeting certain disease categories where we can make the biggest clinical and economic impact. We have to work doubly hard to integrate the elements of care for these afflicted sub-populations. A carefully managed, seamlessly integrated delivery system can most consistently bring the right services and the right information to bear at the right time, all to preserve or improve the membership's over-all health.

For today's vertically integrated delivery systems, this task is prob-ably impossible. Centrally owned and operated systems face tremendous challenges, because they comprise so many different elements with not just conflicting but often competing priorities.

Centrally owned and controlled systems formed just a few years ago are breaking up. Now we are seeing all the hospital-driven foundations, such as Physician Hospital Organizations (PHOs) and poorly functioning Management Service Organizations (MSO), hit the wall that so many pre-dicted they would. Either the physicians or the hospitals reach a point where their losses become too great, and they look to unload. HMOs fi-nally figured out that being in the staff model business and controlling their own delivery network was not the best option. The hospitals face the same scenario, because they cannot enact a broad enough delivery strat-egy; the PHO strategy, where you take everybody on the medical staff and move them into a PHO, just does not work.

A lot of these so-called integrated delivery schemes have been formed not to change the way healthcare is delivered but, rather, to keep managed care at arm's length. They constitute a defensive tactic, not a change strategy. A real-world change strategy first acknowledges that the hospital has to help the managed-care organization take its premiums down from $160 to $100, which means delivering healthcare at $75 for the provider side.

Other industries have abandoned vertical integration in favor of more "virtual" arrangements. Almost every specialized job is out-sourced. When another company can do something better, faster, and cheaper, then let them do it. This more virtual arrangement will proba-bly fare better in healthcare, too. Virtual networks, integrated not by a central power but by mutually beneficial contracts, have become the more relevant model today.

Virtuality excels in its strategic flexibility. The more your fixed costs grow, as they invariably do in a centrally-owned system, the harder it becomes to adjust to the changing marketplace. The well-run virtual network subscribes to the Accordion Theory: it can easily convert its fixed costs to variable costs. Once a virtual network achieves, say, 30 to 50% market share, it can squeeze the accordion, return to a tightly owned system, and then concentrate on getting more efficient and keeping customer service up.

From the outside, such flexible systems might still appear to be vertically integrated, but they are not. Some pieces may be commonly owned, but doctors are free to do what they wish in competition with other doctors, and hospitals are free to do what they wish in competition with other hospitals and HMOs. Only contracts hold the system together. Business is shared among the virtually integrated entities, but always at the going market rates.

Virtual networks are winning the favor of the investment community. When it comes to raising capital, the public markets look askance at organizations that do not employ a financial strategy of owning less and managing more revenues. Having to earn more to get more revenue is not in vogue on Wall Street. Everyone talks about how very capital-intensive system formation is. In fact, access to capital funding is only an issue during the acquisition phase and, to a lesser degree, in purchasing information systems. Healthcare systems are no longer investing in bricks and mortar, where the real big capital dollars used to be spent.

The last thing in the world we need is to watch yet another classic institution topple. We must remind ourselves that integration is not the ultimate goal of the managed-care movement but, rather, an ethereal vehicle by which the business of managing health can best be carried out. Contrary to popular belief, integrating the delivery system, in and of itself, will not accomplish the market reforms we should be enacting by managing population health. When you go into a community and allow everybody to commit to your integrated delivery system, all of the imbalances in that healthcare community will be reflected in your system.

Yet integration has become an absolute prerequisite of managed care. Health plans, for example, have almost no contact with or influence over patient care rendered in physician offices, clinics, or hospitals. The plan's only leverage is via some watered-down incentives concerning member satisfaction. That is not a very positive influence; it is quite

perverse, really. If the way you influence member satisfaction is by joining hands with your physician partners, you had both better be after the
same thing. Either you both believe you will make lots of money through
the partnership or you both believe the job is not about making money.
The "deal" by which the plan and the physicians integrate becomes
the means by which the system can continue to improve the health of a
community.

Speaking of physicians, consider one of the major stumbling blocks
the delivery integrators will soon have to surmount. Today's hordes of internal medicine subspecialists constitute the biggest fudge factor in our
consolidating markets. I am afraid integrated delivery systems will suffer
the consequences of our ludicrous medical overtraining in the 1960s and
1970s. Whenever I speak before the planners of a so-called integrated delivery system, I put two questions to them: (1) What resources will you
need to assemble to serve this population? and (2) How are you going to
get rid of all these specialists?

I say the only way you can truly integrate the delivery system is by,
in effect, forming a classic holding company. There can be no Most
Favored Nation arrangements, transfer pricing, or any of that nonsense.
Each of healthcare's three main lines of business, that is insurance, physician, and facility has to stand on its own legs in the marketplace but the
profits should be measured at the holding company level. The next chapter has much more to say about this thesis of mine.

The Emergence of Provider-based HMO Competition

The number of HMOs operating in the United States reached approximately 600 by mid-1995. About two-thirds of those HMOs are provider-
sponsored. Recent legislation has allowed for provider groups, including
doctors and hospitals, to create health plans called "community health
plans" that will compete directly with HMOs and insurance companies.

Maryland, in March 1996, was the first state to approve a bill em-
powering its legislature to regulate community health networks, which
will contract directly with employers to provide healthcare. The insurer,
however, is not completely eliminated; they may still be necessary to perform certain administrative functions, such as processing claims.
Although these networks are similar to HMOs, they are not required to
meet financial solvency and consumer protection requirements as stringent as those that apply to HMOs.

Medicare Privatization

Although conventional Medicare programs still cover the majority of the elderly, HMOs are being lured into the Medicare coverage arena. The federal government offers generous payments and a large population for those who would manage eldercare. HMOs entering this market have been vying for the business by offering new services, lower prices, and more preventive care. Free health club memberships, zero premiums, zero deductibles, and nonacute drug benefits are among the attractive options HMOs offer to our nation's senior citizens.

Managed-care penetration into the Medicare populations of mature markets seems to be leveling off at about 60 to 65%. The federal government is watching closely to see if managed care is successful in cutting "fat" from the healthcare system and curbing the rise in Medicare spending. Price wars (on supplemental premiums) among HMOs for this business are cropping up in certain regions of the country, as many HMOs are reaping profits ranging from 2 to 5%. Cost cutting via utilization control seems to be the major driver of these profits. The Health Care Financing Administration (HCFA) has seen no proof yet of the promised savings because, in the competition to attract new members, HMOs are providing greater health benefits than required under Medicare legislation. Also yet to be determined is whether the quality of care and overall health status of senior citizens has been affected by the introduction of managed care, or whether HMOs overall have attracted a younger, healthier population.

24-hour Coverage

Managed care is being used throughout the continuum of care, from traditional health services to dental care. Worker's compensation is among the latest service offerings being developed by managed-care companies. In fact, combining medical coverage with worker's compensation has been a recent trend for managed care and insurance companies alike. This combination of medical and worker's compensation coverage, serving members at home and at work, has been referred to as "24-hour coverage."

Employers who believe managed care has helped lower their healthcare costs fervently, hope to reap similar savings in their worker's compensation programs. And if insurers are able to provide comprehensive services under 24-hour coverage, an employer can deal with one carrier for all of its employees' healthcare needs. Applying the concepts of managed care to worker's compensation, insurers believe they can deliver more efficient care and potentially reduce the cost of coverage for occupational medicine.

Managing Image, Reputation, and Financial Strength

With the sharper focus on insurers' accountability for quality of care to recipients, employers, employees, and insurers has come a new focus on managing the market's perception of quality. Accreditation by the National Committee for Quality Assurance (NCQA) has become a widely acknowledged benchmark in this arena.

NCQA accreditation reviews, performed by request or by voluntary application from HMOs, evaluate and rate the quality of healthcare delivery. HMOs can receive "full" accreditation (three years), one-year accreditation, or "provisional" accreditation. HMOs can also fail, which will surely mean lost business in the future. HMOs all over the country are preparing and applying for NCQA accreditation. Other measures of quality being used by payors include customer satisfaction surveys and board certification of physicians.

As the NCQA accreditation process becomes increasingly popular, certain employers (for example, IBM) have taken to offering their employees a shorter menu of exclusively NCQA-accredited HMOs. Xerox and GTE offer financial incentives, in the form of reduced healthcare costs, to employees selecting HMOs with high-quality ratings.

Also under the direction of the NCQA is a set of healthcare measures intended to get the nation's healthcare payors to provide demonstrated value for their customers. Referred to as the Health Plan Employer Data and Information Set (HEDIS), this set of 60 measures are meant to track performance and include reviews of financial stability, clinical performance, access to care, and customer satisfaction. The measures are reported and compiled by HEDIS and made available to the general public. Approximately 300 HMOs and other health plans already use HEDIS. HEDIS continues to modify and expand upon additional areas of measurement, including Medicare and Medicaid services.

Recently, A. M. Best began to rate HMOs, adding them to their historical focus on insurance entities. Basing their involvement on the significant role managed care plays in the healthcare insurance industry today, the potential for ongoing healthcare reform, and the rapid growth in the HMO industry in both enrollment and geographic coverage, A. M. Best introduced its first financial ratings of HMOs in 1995. Intended to provide an opinion on an HMO's financial strength, including operating performance and the ability to meet obligations to the membership, Best's rating system examines an HMO's corporate structure, management objectives, competitive conditions, provider relationships, utilization skills, demographic information, variety of products, pricing strategies, expansion and acquisition strategies, and exposure to state and federal reforms.

Although A. M. Best previously considered HMOs when reviewing and rating their insurance parents, the growing presence of HMOs in the market has moved Best to review HMOs specifically. Consumers, employee benefits managers, and brokers, as well as the HMOs themselves, are supportive of the agency's move. To date, Best's HMO rating process has been voluntary, but all HMOs are likely to join in. High ratings by the reputable agency could instantly differentiate a plan from its competitors and provide a means to communicate operational information, such as long-term plans and management objectives, to the public. Agency ratings may eventually become a market necessity.

Along with NCQA accreditation and A. M. Best ratings, HMOs can also obtain federal qualification. Federal qualification is required for HMOs pursuing Medicare risk contracts. Currently, only about 10% of the Medicare population is served through HMOs. To obtain federal qualification an HMO must satisfy two requirements: (1) it must meet certain provisions of the Public Health Service Act and (2) it must comply with all Medicare standards administered by HCFA.

Globalization and International Ventures

So many of our American originals enjoy their greatest popularity in foreign lands, such as jazz, cigarettes, and Jerry Lewis. So, too, the demand for American healthcare expertise abroad, specifically managed-care expertise, has been increasing as government-run insurance programs overseas are seemingly headed for bankruptcy. Our managed-care industry is being examined as a possible solution to healthcare issues in the global market.

As the cost of healthcare rises in Europe, the rate of healthcare inflation has outpaced the gross domestic product growth since 1990. Certain European nations are looking to shift the risk of healthcare to employers, insurers, and providers. Other factors driving international opportunities for American managed-care companies include the rise of a European middle class, which can afford to spend more on its own healthcare. Population aging is more pronounced in Europe, where approximately 15 to 17% of the population is over 65 years old. In the United States, seniors constitute about 12% of the population.

The sheer infancy of managed care in the overseas markets and the tidal wave of foreigners coming to the United States, for medical expertise and treatments not available in their home countries, may indicate a global market rich with opportunity. But the likelihood that insurers in the United States can succeed in reducing medical costs overseas, despite possible resistance from foreign physicians and public perceptions that quality of care might be adversely affected, must be considered carefully by insurers who endeavor to export their managed-care expertise. Still, as managed care has helped to slow healthcare spending in the United States, providers overseas generally have grown to agree they can use our experiences, not only to shorten their learning curve, but also to improve their ability to provide quality care and improve access to care for populations in need.

OPERATING ISSUES

A number of operating issues will help shape the managed-care market, including changes in the following:

- Insurer strategies;
- Healthcare coalitions;
- Physician incentives;
- Provider network management;
- Information technology;
- Outsourcing practices;
- Capital allocation;
- Capital market access; and
- Healthcare fraud.

Monitoring trends in these areas will yield important information about the immediate future of managed care.

Insurers Sharpen Their Strategic Focus

Mounting competitive pressures are forcing insurers to ask themselves, What business do we really want to be in? Today, insurers must better understand who their customers and competitors are and then focus management on the most strategically significant businesses.

This sharper strategic focus has prompted a number of insurance companies to sell off books of business or entire operating units whose lines of business were not deemed in keeping with the chief mission of the company. In addition, companies have begun to look inward to determine their strongest and weakest functions. Weaker functions, some are just now realizing, can be executed more profitably in other ways. In this light, many insurers have either exited the healthcare arena or joined forces with HMO and other managed-care companies to become dominant forces in the industry.

Mature managed-care markets may be the healthcare insurer's most reliable fortune tellers. An exemplary mature market is Minneapolis/St. Paul, where in essence, if not entirely, a particular set of delivery capabilities is associated with one health plan or a specific financing mechanism. In true managed-care, the physicians' and hospitals' interests are the insurer's interests, too. There is more concern for patients, not less. Once financial incentives and financing mechanisms are aligned to improve the health of the membership, an insurer can help integrate care delivery around its own member advocacy role and the physician's and hospital's patient advocacy role.

Employer Coalitions Drive Quality, Cost Requirements

Healthcare purchasing coalitions in several states have successfully reduced healthcare costs to their member groups, while demanding and receiving improved quality service from their payors. Once feared by the health benefits payors, such coalitions have grown quite popular among employers in Minnesota, Wisconsin, New Jersey, and elsewhere as they have proven their effectiveness.

Most purchasing coalitions contract directly with select payors and impose stringent quality requirements, such as practice guidelines for payors, and mechanisms to track and publish expenditure and utilization data. The larger groups, serving in excess of 700,000 covered lives at large employers, have been able to reduce rates for their members by double-digit percentages simply by bargaining for reduced premiums and specialized products. In scrambling to retain the vast memberships, these coalitions represent payors and providers alike, find themselves with less and less bargaining power in the healthcare marketplace.

Physician Bonuses and Incentives

Typically, bonus incentive programs put physicians at risk by penalizing them if they do not meet or beat budgeted costs. Again, the prime managed-care incentive is to improve health, not cut costs. Managed-care organizations are redefining the typical physician incentive program to focus on quality instead of quantitative indicators of performance. HMOs today wield incentive tools, for example, using generic drugs, using specialists only when necessary, and limiting inpatient stays to align the physicians' interests with the insurer's. The development and refinement of physician-driven, health-oriented incentive programs will be a major force in the managed-care movement.

Provider Networks Shape Local Markets

The competitive nature of the healthcare provider market sets health insurance apart from other insurance products. The strength, reach, and desirability of local provider networks drive competition with other networks for market share. The contracting process with local providers and insurers is the ultimate determinant of price, the other key competitive driver.

Providers, as a group, can still make or break the success of a local network. During employer open enrollment periods, when employees determine if they want to enroll in a different health plan or remain with their current providers, the strength of the participating provider network in the local area and the proportion of the cost members must pay (per visit and as premium) guide the employees' choice of a health plan.

Recent rulings by the United States Justice Department, viewed favorably by the insurance and managed-care companies, have included a rejection of the formation of several large physician networks. The Justice Department, in its ruling, claimed that these deals would violate antitrust laws by placing the network in a position to dictate the terms of arrangements with payors. The department based its decision on verbal testimony by providers who argued that objectives of the network included "obtaining and exercising enhanced bargaining power" in health plan negotiations. The Federal Trade Commission and the Justice Department have pledged to issue new antitrust guidelines for provider networks soon.

Advances in Information Technology

While quality customer service has been a significant focus for insurance and managed-care companies alike, most are only beginning to fulfill their promises. Recent innovations such as on-line enrollment and policy changes, including primary care doctor selection and adding of beneficiaries, have led a rapid flight to technological powerhouses. Electronic networks can now link not only the insurer and the customers, but also competitors, hospitals, physicians, pharmacies, billing companies, third-party administrators, and ambulance companies. Commonly referred to in the industry as community health information networks (CHINs), these healthcare equivalents of the automated teller machine offer all participants in the health system the ability to communicate through a shared network via common interfaces. Few payors have done significant research into the value of CHINs to the consumer (and the financial benefits to themselves), and even fewer have invested the millions necessary to develop them.

Most indemnity insurers rely on a variety of legacy systems of antique vintage. Managed-care companies tend to have newer but less sophisticated systems. Both payor groups are beginning to realize that old and new systems are not providing the array of information needed to effectively manage the business. Unfortunately, the cost of upgrading or changing a system is often prohibitive. CHINs may provide a useful solution for the future, as they require no replacement of systems that already work well but, rather, a mere enhancement of connections and a few new built-in systems to allow for electronic transfer.

Despite the many challenges, CHINs are being developed in all fifty states, most still at the single-enterprise level. CHIN proponents note that they provide unprecedented 24-hour on-line access to medical information, reduce administrative costs (specifically "paper trails"), and increase billing accuracy. CHIN opponents say that data security and patient confidentiality, as well as political issues, outweigh the advantages. Costs could also become an issue, as fees to join the network are high, as are one-time software costs and monthly fees for physicians. Besides, since many of the systems presently in use at managed-care and indemnity-health insurance companies are proprietary, broad participation in a shared network may be precluded in many communities.

Outsourcing

As competition in the managed-care and health-insurance industries heats up to a boil, companies large and small face critical decisions to make or buy the services and expertise their enrollees need. Outsourcing financial and administrative services, often including but not limited to claims processing, premium billing and collection, information technology, and internal audit, may allow a company to achieve desired profitability and efficiency. Employees, in many cases, can still be retained by the outsourcing entity.

Outsourcing is emblematic of our Age of Specialization. Employers, seeing outsourcing as a means to control rising costs of providing services, give the external contractor responsibility for managing one or more services. Because it specializes in providing a particular service, the contractor may be able to provide that service more efficiently and less expensively than the insurer. An outsourcing insurer can concentrate more effectively on its core businesses.

Capital Allocation Strategies

Capital is a limited resource that insurers must deploy carefully, and hospitals and physician groups must be more careful yet. Dwindling profit margins, increased competition (from both traditional and nontraditional sources), rising capital requirements among regulators and rating agencies, slow to moderate growth in many segments in which insurers compete are all these trends that make capital deployment decisions critical today.

Managed-care enterprises may need to craft a capital allocation strategy (1) when deciding how best to invest capital resources and (2) to continuously monitor/analyze capital allocation decisions against other deployment alternatives. A sound capital allocation strategy:

- Seeks to allocate scarce capital resources among alternatives to maximize enterprise profits, sustain growth and strategic advantages, and manage risk;
- Helps an insurer focus resources toward the most profitable and promising opportunities and away from less promising alternatives;
- Is integrated with an insurer's overall strategic plans and reflects the enterprise's risk posture and financial goals; and
- Guides the enterprise to invest resources where the expected return is commensurate with the enterprise's overall strategy, financial objectives, and appetite for risk, then provides a mechanism to monitor progress toward these objectives.

Formulating a thoughtful capital allocation strategy is perhaps the single most important action an insurer can take to develop and maintain a future competitive advantage.

Access to Capital Markets

Capital is a scarce resource for which health insurers and managed-care companies compete with all other insurance and noninsurance enterprises, such as all the physician and hospital corporations in the recent flood of independent public offerings. The ability to access capital is critical to the successful growth and prosperity of health insurers, particularly given the rising requirements of regulators and rating agencies. Health insurers with successful strategies for attracting and utilizing capital resources will have a distinct advantage in the marketplace.

A health insurer's access to various capital markets is largely a function of its ability to differentiate itself from competitors through a knowledge of capital markets, successful corporate strategies, effective capital allocation strategies, and other ingredients that mark bright prospects for ongoing success.

Healthcare Fraud

As the pressures increase on healthcare providers and consumers, concerns mount about potential fraud and the potential impact of fraudulent acts. From providers miscoding diagnoses and procedures to consumers submitting claims simultaneously under health insurance and worker's compensation policies, fraud is an everyday occurrence that insurers work hard to prevent.

Software is playing an ever increasing role in testing for unbundling of codes and for consistency of diagnosis. Computers are also helping many companies detect patterns of behavior among providers that may indicate the overutilization of certain procedures. Publicity about varying rates for cesarean sections, for example, has brought more attention to providers' use of that procedure. Of course overutilization does not always indicate fraud, but a number of heavily publicized cases of system abuse, particularly in the Medicare arena, have been brought to light by tracking overutilization of selected procedures.

REGULATORY ISSUES

Some say a camel is just a horse designed by a committee, and more than a few would say our healthcare system owes its pronounced oddities to the absurd machinations of bureaucrats. Certainly the market watcher should follow regulatory affairs in the following key areas:

- National healthcare reform;
- Medicare and Medicaid reforms;
- State managed-care regulations;
- Market conduct; and
- Not-for-profit versus for-profit HMO status.

Good luck figuring out what all those politicians and appointees might do before they do it. And do trust that market reform will long remain the stronger wave of change to monitor.

National Healthcare Reform

As a result of continued political changes in Washington, epitomized by the Republicans gaining control of the House of Representatives and Senate in 1995, national healthcare reform was effectively defeated. With this defeat the harsh spotlight on providers of healthcare (and the high cost of providing care) was effectively dimmed and, as a result, both medical costs and utilization rates may be set to skyrocket.

Although the future for national healthcare reform is uncertain in Washington, it continues to be a topic of budget debates and a prime consideration among United States' citizens and state and federal legislators. As more Americans confront difficulties relating to the availability, affordability, and portability of healthcare coverage, reform of the healthcare system seems imminent but may be years off.

Medicare and Medicaid Reform Packages

For the past several years, both the House and the Senate have plastered us with proposals that could mean significant financial and structural changes in the Medicare and Medicaid spending programs. Savings achieved from cuts in these programs are believed to be the key to achieving a balanced budget, a principle to which both the Executive and Legislative branches have committed. But because the federal government is really discussing managed *financing,* as opposed to managed *care,* total Medicare and Medicaid spending is anticipated to grow between 5 and 6% annually, even while costs decline in the commercial sector.

Of primary interest to insurers is the future role of managed care for the nation's senior citizens. Recently proposed Medicare bills promise a solution to the anticipated bankruptcy of this program by the year 2002 and, as a result, continue to force the Medicare market transition from indemnity to managed care. These bills additionally threaten to eliminate certain antitrust laws, providing opportunity for additional provider-run health plans. Competition for the Medicare members will intensify competition among insurers and providers and increase the risk of depressed profit margins in Medicare managed-care products.

HMO incentive programs, now effective in most states, reduce the risk of each state's Medicaid program (state-level healthcare coverage for welfare recipients) and transfer some of this risk to the HMOs. Rather than being reimbursed on a fee-for-service basis, the states set up programs where HMOs get capitated rates to accept responsibility for the care of Medicaid recipients. Medicaid patients benefit in gaining access to an active physician network rather than having to seek care themselves. The states benefit through reduced medical risks and administrative costs.

Managed-care companies continue to scramble for Medicaid business. According to the HCFA home page, in 1995 about 28% (11.6 million) of our nation's 41.4 million Medicaid eligibles were enrolled in some type of managed-care program. Regulation related to Medicaid continues at the state level. The nation's governors continue their sponsorship of a Medicaid reform bill that would overhaul certain components of the current Medicaid program and includes provisions to reduce federal and state matching fund rates, to change the way federal funding of the program is distributed, and to reduce the amount states would have to pay into the program.

Other significant proposed changes include reducing the duration and level of benefits provided (with a "floor" put in place) and limiting the rights of providers to sue states in federal court over benefits and reimbursement rates.

Also, part of the proposed Medicare bills and the balanced budget amendments are medical savings accounts (MSAs). Taxpayers choosing to funnel pretax dollars into a MSA would be eligible for a high-deductible, low-premium health insurance policy. Unused amounts at the end of the year would revert to the employee, creating incentives for more cost-conscious personal medical spending. Fewer than 2000 employers in the United States used MSAs as of early 1996; only seven states have enacted MSA legislation. Critics believe that MSAs may also cause employees to avoid preventive care in order to reserve the cost. Others claim only the young and healthy will select MSAs, thus potentially driving up healthcare costs of the nation.

State-Level Managed Care Regulations

In the absence of a national reform package, many states have passed healthcare reform legislation of their own. Certain states have mandated 48-hour hospital stays for maternity cases, while others have dealt with the issues of improving availability and affordability of health insurance to small employers, eliminating exclusions for preexisting conditions, instituting the guaranteed renewal of healthcare, and ensuring the easy portability of healthcare coverage from employer to employer or unemployment.

The state of Washington has been leading one so-called anti-managed care campaign, taking 48-hour maternity stays to another level altogether; a mandatory-stay bill that would bar insurers and HMOs from setting any limits on maternity and newborn inpatient stays is awaiting approval by the governor of Washington. Other state legislation bills include the "any willing provider" initiative, which requires that physicians meeting minimum contract requirements may not be excluded from the panel of physicians in a managed-care organization. The goal is to provide individuals with the greatest possible choice of doctors. Managed-care organizations have opposed the bill as contrary to the concept of controlling cost by posting the primary care physician as a system gatekeeper. But the final question is, Who will pay for more luxury of choice?

Market Conduct

Market conduct remains a top issue in the insurance industry, including insurance department-regulated HMOs, and has received attention as a rating issue (by A. M. Best) that can affect a company's financial and competitive position.

Market conduct examinations focus on sales and marketing practices, including distribution channels, and are conducted by state insurance departments.

The National Association of Insurance Commissioners (NAIC) has adopted Market Conduct Guidelines that describe minimum laws and regulations a state should have to address unfair trade practices and examination authority. The NAIC continues to work on the process for coordinating multistate market conduct examinations. The association has also developed an extensive coordinated database network to facilitate the sharing of information between states about regulatory investigations of improper sales and marketing practices of companies and agents.

Not-for-Profit versus For-Profit HMO Status

Another regulatory issue on the horizon is being addressed by the Internal Revenue Service (IRS). Nearly since the inception of managed care, the IRS has been skeptical about the justification for tax-exempt status for nonprofit HMOs and, furthermore, confused about whether certain activities, such as providing point-of-service products, should disqualify an HMO of its nonprofit status. Currently, approximately 70% of the nation's nearly 600 health maintenance organizations operate as for-profit entities.

One of the major reasons for selecting for-profit status for an HMO is the differences in access to capital. As the competition intensifies for capital to foster growth, the ability to obtain capital will become a critical success factor. More and more, the bond market is a nonprofit organization's only means for raising capital.

S U M M A R Y

It should be obvious from a quick scan of the economic, social, market, operating, and regulatory issues discussed in this chapter, managed care has become interwoven with the very fabric of our national life. One hesitates to echo the infamous boast that what is good for managed care is good for America, or vice versa. But is it too early to say that managed care is our best bet for high-quality, universally accessible, and easily affordable healthcare? It is a rhetorical question at this late date. Insurers, providers, physicians, governments, employers, and consumers have embraced the managed-care concept and no doubt will see to its future growth.

Which brings us to the heart of the matter: How far along are we, where should we be going, and how can we get there? All the ambitious managed-care champion needs now is a shiny new conceptual framework by which everyone can view the present and future healthcare marketplace. Observed in proper perspective, the mysterious competitive behaviors and somewhat disruptive episodes of recent times might be more clearly understood as either inconsequential skirmishes, which we can safely ignore, or necessary passages to a brighter future, which we can and must endure. The next chapter constructs just such a framework.

3

CHAPTER

The Managed-Care Pinwheel—A New Conceptual Framework

The American disease, said a brilliant someone whose name escapes me, is forgetfulness. How quickly we forget what made our nation the world leader in healthcare. And how quick we are to discard perfectly fine working arrangements in favor of half-baked ideas and wholly unworkable schemes. Managed care must neither forget nor discard the past successes of American healthcare but, to accomplish a worthwhile and lasting change, must build anew upon its strongest pillars. Those pillars stand firm today.

Our nation and our healthcare industry can boast a century of progress that has witnessed the construction of an enviable system of public health, still second to none, still rather neatly divided into the following three main sectors:

1. Hospitals, run with the operational discipline of crack military units, outfitted with the most sophisticated equipment and supplies, and covering the broadest possible range of health needs and localities, from community acute care hospitals, to regional tertiary facilities, to national specialty clinics, and to world-renowned academies;

2. Payors, led by profitable insurance companies and generously funded federal and state social endowments; and

3. <u>Physicians</u>, bound in a proud fraternity of plentiful supply constantly replenished by the best medical schools, constantly informed by the strongest research core, and constantly supported by the brightest nursing and technical professionals.

Add to this mix our nation's fine legacy of beneficent employers, labor unions, professional associations, charitable foundations, and retirement plans, and it all equals a veritable embarrassment of healthcare riches. Our healthcare system has grown up so big and strong because, until quite recently, each of the three main sectors has built intently upon the bedrock of its special experiences, knowledge, and expertise; hospitals delivered care, payors insured populations, and physicians practiced medicine.

Suddenly, everyone wants to own and control everyone else's enterprise. Physicians dabble in hospital ownership, insurance dabble in physician ownership, hospitals dabble in physician group management. I call it the "Last Waltz of the Dinosaurs," because all these dabblings and entanglements are really the death spasms of a species soon to be extinct. Few of the mergers or affiliations between payor, physician, and provider entities have been founded on a vision to truly manage care or integrate delivery. With all this sound and fury, signifying nothing, we may be squandering our chances for meaningful change and forward progress.

I contend our brightest hope is our surest strength. Whatever else has transpired since managed care first made its splash in the market, and whatever exciting advancements the future might yet hold in store, some things will not, should not and cannot change.

THE CASE FOR A NEW CONCEPTUAL FRAMEWORK

Healthcare must forever comprise very different businesses run by very different people. Insurers, providers, and doctors bring distinctive viewpoints, interests, and contributions to a healthcare community long held stable by a system of checks and balances. This sensitive balance serves the public good. Recently, though, guided less by concerns for public health and more by ambition and greed, the marketplace seems to have become a whirlwind bent on razing every classic institution, every tradition, good or ill. Some believe the divisible industry sectors will soon relinquish their self-reliant control and ownership to a new breed of *managed-care organization,* a name as roundly misunderstood as managed care itself.

We continue along this course at our peril. Payors, providers, and physicians had better stop swapping properties and start exchanging information and ideas that contribute to the common cause of health improvement. Somehow we must keep the industry segmented but not fragmented. Segmentation makes sense when staking out a manageable span of system ownership and control, but fragmentation in the care delivery continuum has become an intolerable threat to the health of our communities.

What is now a blur of market activity may soon come to rest, or very nearly so. A more sensible conceptual framework ought to emerge in sharp focus, as the managed care industry matures, marketplace by marketplace. Sometimes such a clarifying image needs a little coaxing.

Making plain sense of all the powers at work in today's managed-care marketplace is quite a taxing proposition. Capturing that sense whole, in a single graphic image, may be altogether impossible. For one thing, we endeavor to view not one homogenous managed-care marketplace but many diverse local healthcare financing and delivery systems at once. So we should not toy with static scale models, shrink-wrapped and packaged with molded part trees and easy-to-follow assembly directions. Instead we should concern ourselves with plotting dynamic orbits of association and spheres of influence and, ultimately, should express our findings in terms of managed care's unstoppable inertia: the driving rotational and organizing centripetal forces already shaping a new era in American healthcare.

All this may sound like a pompous buildup for a notion as silly as a pinwheel. But make no mistake, this Managed Care Pinwheel is serious marketplace physics, if you want, call it a propeller beanie. The pinwheels we know are cheap, plentiful, and disposable novelties. This is not so for the managed care pinwheel. But this pinwheel does spin wildly with every forward motion, capturing and displaying the winds of change while perhaps teaching an important lesson in elementary market aerodynamics. One uncommonly visual colleague of mine can not seem to shake the image of portly men riding tiny tricycles, sporting red fezzes, and a shiny foil pinwheel twirling on each set of handlebars. A fitting enough image, I say.

INTRODUCING THE PINWHEEL

Figure 3–1, The Managed-Care Pinwheel, illustrates the future managed-care marketplace I envision. To me, this figure represents the culmination of managed care's promising trajectory from (a) a shifting cluster of members-only enterprises into (b) a reliable, communitywide system of competitive but cooperative payors and providers who are jointly and severally responsible for monitoring, managing, and improving population health. A pinwheel-like market configuration allows each industry sector to wield its trademark strengths but discourages any tampering with the critical integrating forces, namely case management techniques, community health records, and shared information technologies, which occupy the pinwheel's hub.

In other words, the managed-care pinwheel, not coincidentally, embodies our familiar motif. Only the free exchange of intellectual capital through advanced information technology and case management techniques, all with a sharp eye toward better health outcomes, will keep managed care moving in the right direction.

Parts and Functions

The managed-care pinwheel has three blades folded to form a Möbius strip, which represents the full continuum of care and the full spectrum of entities by which care is financed and delivered. In short, one pinwheel portrays one comprehensive, integrated healthcare network, including the following:

- Payors offering the entire range of insurance products, from self-insurance and traditional indemnity to HMOs, point-of-service plans, and PPOs, any of which may practice a lite to heavy application of managed-care techniques;
- Clinicians of all backgrounds and disciplines, including nurse practitioners and other ancillary providers as well as primary-care doctors and physician specialists, subspecialists, and superspecialists; and
- Providers based in bricks-and-mortar facilities or serving scattered sites along the continuum of care from wellness, social services, and home health to subacute, acute, intensive care, and beyond, including transplants and other tertiary care services.

The pinwheel makes visual the mounting forces of integration within and between these traditional industry sectors. At the fastening hub resides the system's shared intellectual capital investments, such as strong case management programs, advanced information technologies, and permanent community health records by which these traditional industry sectors can integrate delivery, financing, and, ultimately, manage population health.

The basic assumption behind the managed-care pinwheel is that capital sharing among system entities, merely for the sake of capturing one

Managed-care organizations, physicians, or hospital systems can serve as managed-care integrators or vendors. Intellectual capital is at the core of successful integration, primarily in the form of information systems, case management, and health records.

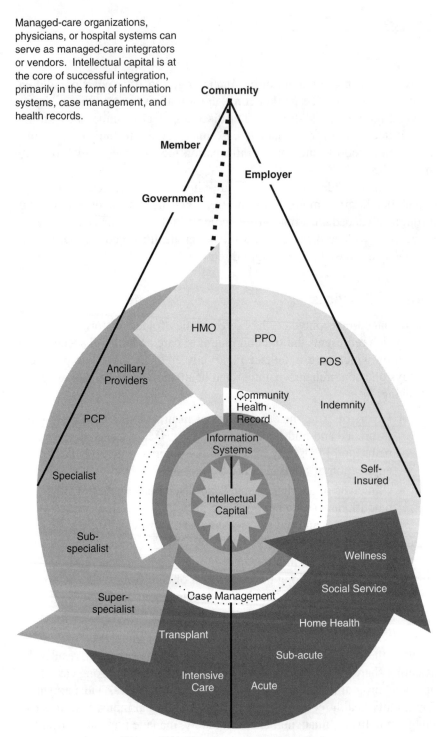

Figure 3–1   The Managed-Care Pinwheel

another's businesses, will not create the financing and delivery model we should desire. The current wave of hospitals, physicians, and insurance companies using their precious capital dollars to acquire and operate other parts of the system does not, in my view, make a lot of sense. The appropriate goal is not to outsmart or outmuscle your partners across your own pinwheel but, rather, to orchestrate a meeting of minds and create solidarity in the managed population health movement.

PINWHEELS IN MOTION TODAY

Every day my reading reveals another piece of evidence in support of the general managed-care pinwheel theory. Following just one example, I have watched the Advocate Health Care system, serving metropolitan Chicago, divest of its health plan business to focus on being the best provider network it can be. "We are in a market that has relatively mature managed-care plans, and it would be too strong a capital commitment for us to be competitive," the Advocate's president and CEO has been quoted. "We do not have access to the stock market like others. We want to continue to focus on rounding out our network and continuing to be a good provider."*

This is an enlightened strategic stance in a market that has become so preoccupied with expansion and acquisition. In tapping the strength of its roots and remembering the roots of its strength, Advocate has begun building a managed-care pinwheel that will better serve the health of its community. The system did indeed sell its plan, to Humana, for more than $20 million.**

As I see it, pinwheels have been in full swing for several years, while most observers have been more fascinated by the admittedly more fascinating cross-industry mergers and acquisitions. We should be less concerned about transferring money and more concerned about shuttling plan members, scientific and business data, and medical knowledge across the hub of the system.

Propelling New Market Behaviors

In healthcare, as elsewhere, the grass is always greener on the other side. Those Joneses across the street are hogging all the money and having all the fun. And they are forever leaning over the fence gossiping about you,

---

*"Advocate system to sell health plan," *Modern Healthcare,* 22 April 1996, p. 33.
**"Humana to buy Advocate unit," *Modern Healthcare,* 13 January 1997, p. 16.

no doubt with the Smiths next door, or planning another party you will not be invited to, or having another good laugh at your expense. The essentially cooperative business of integrated, managed population healthcare cannot abide such unneighborly market behaviors.

Pinwheel thinking encourages market behaviors that foster rather than undermine the managed-care movement. An organization that concentrates on the part of the system it knows so well and then works to handle all aspects of that industry, without digressing to wield capital dollars and acquire organizations it has no business owning and operating, will actually fare much better in a managed-care environment. One might call this the "Right What You Know" school of managed care.

But for the whole system to be effective, for the good of its members and of the community, all parties must also share certain information and resources. Essential integrating elements include good case management (managing members' care, not patients' movement), a common repository of medical records (community-based, not patient-based), and shared information systems and technologies that allow parties to exchange information without necessarily exchanging capital.

The pinwheel is not a static model of the market. In managed-care lite markets, several pinwheels may intersect at various points, more like cogs meshing together. As a market matures and consolidates, two or three major pinwheels dominate. Yet new pinwheels may emerge at any time, as new players with new products enter the market. By contract or partnership, each pinwheel can assemble any number of payor, provider, and physician entities. A well-crafted pinwheel then becomes the chief integrating and competing unit, vying to outperform and outintegrate the other pinwheels forming in the marketplace.

SHARING INTELLECTUAL CAPITAL—AT THE PINWHEEL'S HUB

If the managed-care pinwheel is the new unit of integration and competition, then shared intellectual capital is the hub that holds the pinwheeled system together and perpetually revolving about the common focus of health. Payors, providers, and physicians alike must sacrifice essential elements of their autonomy to the healthcare community as a whole and to the mission of population health management. All must acknowledge that certain assets and functions rightly belong to the system as a whole. Former weapons of competition must become the new means of collaboration between payor, provider, and physician organizations.

Foremost among the items of intellectual capital every managed care community must share are the following:

- Seamless *case management* programs that guide individual members along the most clinically effective and economically efficient course from diagnosis, through quality care processes, and back to health;
- Member *health records* that permanently reside in a secure but accessible community repository; and
- Powerful *information systems* that speed the analysis of population and comparative data for epidemiologic study.

The highest aspirations of payors, physicians, and providers will come to nothing if we cannot put these core elements in place at the very center of every American healthcare community. Here our investment in managed care and population health management must begin.

Case Management

Our application of proven case management techniques needs to go much deeper and much wider. A "case" never begins with a member's contraction of an acute or chronic illness. Case managers must dig deeper into populations at risk and follow up with postcare populations to track outcomes and inform the system's constant clinical, quality, and cost improvements. Nor is managing a "case" the sole responsibility of any one sector of the healthcare community. Too many, indeed some practitioners of the art, misconstrue case management as a payor-imposed system under which a deputized police force sets out to limit services and deny coverage, by any legal means necessary. Pinwheel thinking urges payors, providers, and physicians to cooperate with new and sometimes independently contracted care-managing entities that must help patients bridge the scattered sites and assemble the fragmented continuum of care.

Any number of disciplines may provide qualified case managers. Family members and rank-and-file hospital staff working under the guidance of nursing professionals and social workers may, in fact, prove to be our best case managers yet. Payor-, provider-, or physician-sponsored, the effective case management program will convince each sector that it is working for the common interests of all three. And as in all managed-care endeavors, providing no more and no less case management than is absolutely necessary will strike the right balance for success.

One can easily underestimate the value of one good case manager, who possesses the precious knowledge that doctors, nurses, and consumers themselves used to possess in simpler times. A qualified case manager knows all the clinical, fiscal, social, and community resources at the member's disposal and, more important, knows how best to match those resources with the member's particular needs to achieve the best clinical and economic outcomes. It is as simple as that; and as complex as that.

Community Health Records

Today's scattered medical records must become permanent health records for entire communities of health plan members. When a member visits an institution for the first time or even switches insurance plans, the community health record must remain in place and intact.

Once, when my employer dumped a general PPO in favor of a restricted PPO, dropping my personal doctor in the process, I ended up having to undergo a battery of tests just to establish a baseline record for my new physician. Even though I lived and worked in the same community and for the same firm all that time, my medical history could not be shared. I was fragmented among all the facilities and doctors I had ever visited. The cost and bother of performing the baseline tests is built right into the fragmented delivery system. How much more efficient and manageable it would be to build information sharing into the system.

Granted, the Information Age introduces new legislative worries concerning the confidentiality and security of sensitive data, such as medical records. As we map new frontiers on the imaginary landscape of cyberspace, new rules cannot be far behind. Remember, though, electronic data systems do not inherently lack security, any more than paper records do. It is all a matter of responsible storage and handling. Surely the benefits of community records far outweigh any potential legal drawbacks or technologic hurdles. We will find the way forward, if only after years of vigorous debate and further evidence that security and privacy can be assured.

Information Systems

Sophisticated community health information networks remain frustratingly just beyond our grasp. We have the available information processing and telecommunications technology to establish a smoothly functioning repository of electronic community health records, and other vital health data for epidemiologic study, if only someone would take the responsibility for setting up and operating such systems.

Some new player to the healthcare business may have to step in and pick up the slack. Internet service providers, telephone and cable companies, software publishers, and even entertainment industries may soon rise to the challenge. DreamWorks, for example, is now interconnecting hospitals so sick children can discuss their illnesses on-line with similarly afflicted boys and girls all over the world. The video interface displays cartoons the children create for one another.

In terms of implementing the powerful information systems needed to support strong case management programs and electronic community health records, at least the following three design elements will be critical to success:

1. Friendliness—Clinicians and planners can easily retrieve selected information in a format suited for review and integration with clinical decision support and other systems.

2. Security—System designers must strike the right balance between access and security with passwords, electronic signatures, and enforceable policies and procedures.

3. Flexibility—System technologies and applications must be able to change and grow with a changing and growing pinwheel. Above all, shared information systems must flexibly automate essential case management processes and health record maintenance.*

We will be years and years setting the foundation for community-wide information networks that meet these lofty goals. Major system implementation is a challenge for a single healthcare organization, let alone for several major organizations in a young partnership. Able designers can surely engineer technologies to fit the application. But it will be up to executive leaders and managers to ensure that core processes are also engineered to suit the technologies. Friendly, secure, and flexible information systems are not made so in schematic drawings but in everyday use by everyday people.

---

*After Wakerly, Ralph T., ed., Community Health Information Networks: Creating the Health Care Data Highway (Chicago: American Hospital Publishing, 1994) pp. 28-30.

S U M M A R Y

Strong case management programs, sophisticated information technologies, electronic community health records, which is the hub of the managed-care pinwheel, is really all about communicating better. Payors, physicians, and providers must communicate with one another, more clearly than ever before, to share vital data about the health of plan members who visit caregivers scattered among numerous sites. A core of information must be established and secured, the lines always kept open, and just the right knowledge put at the fingertips of the professional who can make the soundest clinical decision and do the most good for the member.

The managed-care pinwheel represents but one vision of the future healthcare marketplace and that is the singular vision that is mine to share with you. No perfect picture will rush to the visual aid of all concerned parties. Let it be. For the purposes of my argument we can hazard this grand design, this pinwheel. One momentarily shared vision, however silly and imperfect, might allow us to glimpse several likely futures for managed care, as discussed in Chapter 4. Only then can we intelligently discuss and eventually master a new calculus, as explained in the chapters that follow, by which anyone can describe the restless change and constant motion across the industry or in a given marketplace.

4
CHAPTER

Our Managed-Care Trajectory

To borrow the commercial hook from a popular board game, managed care takes just minutes to learn but a lifetime to master. So inspiring are the central themes of managed care, such as its refreshing emphasis on preventing illness and preserving health, its fine balance between clinical excellence and fiscal responsibility, that one might easily underestimate the gargantuan task facing those who would embrace such lofty virtues out here in the real world. Managed care eludes the casual observer. What may seem like common-sense principles are really bold visions. What may seem like basic tools are really tough disciplines. What may seem like an overnight sensation has really been years in the making, and will just as surely be years in the refining.

In fact, as we have observed, managed care has not even arrived yet. But most everyone agrees it is here to stay, most everyone agrees, and most everyone stands at the ready to go. So the healthcare industry news these days reads like another colorful chapter of American history. All the familiar territory having been settled or spoiled, everyone wants to whoop it up on the next wild frontier. Managed-care organizations are doing a land-office business as hospitals and physicians scramble to seize bold new opportunities and fortunes for themselves. Still, prospectors who sniff a jackpot in every dull nugget seem to outnumber the sober practitioners who have troubled to set up viable operations focused on health.

In this chapter we consider some of the critical viewpoints, activities, and proclivities that will shape the future of managed care. The snippets of conversation we eavesdrop upon here have been assembled from my travels and personal meetings with some of managed care's noted luminaries and voices of authority, as well as from the healthcare business literature and other readings. Share with me the viewpoints of members, hospital systems, alternative providers, health plans, physician groups, pharmaceutical houses, and the endangered research and educational core of our healthcare system, the medical academies. Together, these colors and shadings all but complete our sketch of the managed-care landscape, no doubt a work in constant progress.

MEMBERS IN MOTION

The promise of communitywide health management could turn out to be just another healthcare pipe dream if managed-care plans cannot capture a strong majority of lives and keep membership stable. What might urge more people to join up? And what might convince members to remain loyal to a plan? In short, what do people expect of a health plan, and what keeps them healthy, happy, and enrolled?

Image Versus Reality

When I am flying I often complain that if airlines spent as much time training their employees as they do advertising how friendly their employees are, they would probably be better off. When I am driving and see a big billboard advertising some healthcare payor, invariably claiming "We Really Care" complete with a picture of a pregnant woman or an adorable infant, I often complain that if health plans spent as much time improving membership services as they do plastering billboards, they would probably be better off.

Members shop for access, responsiveness, and quality. But the only real choices users have are what plan to join and, perhaps, what primary care physician to use. The rest is 95 percent provider-directed. When you look at an ultracompetitive market like California, all the plans offer pretty much the same doctors and hospitals, and the benefits match up pretty evenly. There is no real differentiation left but price, and that is no real differentiation in most consumers' minds.

Friendly, helpful service might be another better way for health plans to distinguish themselves in a maturing managed-care market. Some 40% of members have zero interaction with the care delivery system in any given year. What if one plan reengineered its membership services department to truly provide membership services instead of just handle complaints? The department could actually make physician appointments and coordinate referrals for members. That might build a more fitting image of quality and friendliness to attract new members and keep current members.

A Lasting Satisfaction

Still, the truest measure of success in managing care is a plan's ability to respond with an honest and resounding "yes" to the question, Are all our members getting the care they need? More than mere gimmickry, a culture built around a genuine concern for the membership makes a health plan go.

In the members-only world of managed care, customer satisfaction is not so important as customer loyalty. Here, loyalty does not mean frequent use of the system but, rather, a lasting commitment to remain a dues-paying member of the health plan. Nothing saps a health plan's bottom line faster than a wave of member disenrollments. Members' active migrations also make it difficult to define and study the population and, ultimately, to manage health.

Customer satisfaction campaigns are the logical place to begin fighting the disenrollment problem. As long as they are being treated fairly and their doctor has an amenable bedside manner, members will likely stay loyal to the plan. Proper incentives for members will keep barriers at a minimum, so people in need of healthcare are not making their initial contact decisions predicated on how much it is going to cost them. No one should be seeking or not seeking care based on the amount of the benefit cap. That would be entirely antithetical to the fundamental principles of managed care.

If members are waiting too long for certain kinds of visits, the responsible, and responsive health plan might deploy nonphysician professionals or implement a new communication and scheduling system. You can not just say, "Look, we are seeing too much utilization here, so we are going to have to impose limits or raise co-payments." The plan struck a deal, remember, to bear a risk for the health of a population. Members will take notice and take to the road should the plan renege on that deal.

HOSPITAL SYSTEMS IN MOTION

I keep waiting for the industry consolidation we have been hearing so much about. For five years in the 1980s I made my living downsizing hospitals. Now here in California among many of the institutions whose financial profiles baffled me back then, most of them are still hanging on, without having changed the way they do business. The underperforming hospitals that finally did close were mostly the little ones out on the fringes.

When you close a hospital and shift its volume to a facility down the street, costs go down, clinical quality and shareholder value go up, and the painful losers are the employees who lose their jobs. Maybe the government should pay some hospitals to shut down, like they pay some farmers not to plow their fields, and help outplace the affected employees. Economically speaking, one could convincingly demonstrate that aggressive consolidation would benefit the community as a whole. I hate to look to the government to solve any problem, but maybe that would speed market-driven reforms along.

The Exploding Hospital

Hospitals, it has been widely predicted, will either become highly efficient Intensive Care Units (ICUs) or go out of business. How will hospital leaders worried about mere survival, play the role of care innovators? Their track record is pretty poor. And virtually every prudent innovation will take patients away from the hospital. What brave administrators will be willing to kill themselves off? Hospital people hold an indelible bias that the hospital is the utmost appropriate place to provide all healthcare.

Our leading hospitals of tomorrow will become centers of health today. They will develop rational networks guided by policies that treat providers fairly but with certain expectations for accountability. Hospitals must grow to view themselves as staunch advocates for the populations they serve, that is the people whose health they help preserve. They will need to get a fix on the defined population, study the group of diseases and conditions that most affect that population, and then develop the wherewithal to truly manage health.

The Exploding Hospital Executive Suite

Hospitals are really going to struggle with the impending transformations. They have got to do a better job of managing costs, as do physicians.

Hospitals should work hardest at getting their costs in order and developing lasting relationships with strong physician companies. We all have to change our behaviors and fundamentally change how healthcare is delivered. These will not be merely financial changes but a profound change in the very business we are in. We are migrating from a sickness business to a health business.

Can today's hospital executive manage such a transformation from the administrative suite? Not likely. Over the past twenty years, our nation's business schools have produced an executive class lacking any real understanding of the epidemiologic principles of public health. A new breed of hospital leader may soon emerge, or new executive skill sets and teams may have to be dreamt up and patched together, like so many monsters in Frankenstein's laboratory.

The hospital is the worst place to end up and everybody knows it. There is much more infection, disease, and harsh light in the hospital than anywhere else in the world. One hospital, in an innocent attempt to claim superiority over its competitors in the area, launched a campaign telling employers how much lower its infection rate was. Employers were shocked at the very mention of such a problem. They had no idea there was such a higher risk of infections in the hospital setting.

Employers and enrollees view hospitalization as the failure of every other possible alternative, and that is the health-oriented viewpoint our entire system should be adopting.

ALTERNATIVE PROVIDERS ON THE MOVE

In managing care, effective provider organizations will learn how to integrate numerous scattered care sites, while carefully aligning sometimes divergent missions and values. Aiming to minimize the use of the hospital, the virtually integrated systems of the future will not tie themselves down to any one physical location or nerve center. Daily medical decisions will rest with care managers who are not attached to any particular physical place. Their only true measures of success and accountability will be what is happening in the population in terms of health status, clinical outcomes, and costs of care.

Perhaps the richest opportunities for alternative providers lie in delivering more care in patients' very own homes and at places of work. Such care might best be delivered not by human visitors but by extremely friendly information systems. Little by little we are handing the reins of our healthcare system over to patients, their families and caregivers, and cable and on-line networks. The computer-savvy, under-50 generation is already hip to this news. We should constantly be surveying the landscape for new patient care tools that get people back home where they belong.

Just like hospital people, many ambulatory care professionals contemplating the home-care movement will cling to their bricks-and-mortar viewpoint. In the minds of administrators, hospital-based physicians, and subspecialists, it is difficult to imagine that any care responsibilities should rightly move from physicians to nonphysicians, from hospitals and ambulatory care facilities to the patient home, or from the healthcare system to the consumer.

Physicians today control upwards of 80% of all healthcare costs. They order virtually all the hospitalizations, the diagnostic tests, the procedures, the therapies, and the drugs. Some estimates claim that physician practices manage about $200 billion but actually control more like $800 billion. And these practices have little information to help them pilot such a vast chunk of our national economy. Doctors do a fine job controlling hospital days. But the other 40% of the institutional pool, mostly Skilled Nursing Facility (SNF) care, is poorly managed. Physicians need to get involved not just in shifting patients out of hospitals and into SNFs, but also in looking hard at what constitutes appropriate care and a reasonable length of stay once a patient arrives at the SNF or other alternative site. More and more, the patient's own home is the clinically and economically preferable care setting. Sounder choices of care settings can only be driven by sounder information in the hands of physicians.

We have never seen the likes of this era, this genuine industrialization of medicine. What is going to happen to hospitals? What is most likely to take their place? I am not sure if anybody has the right answer, exactly. But the surgery center, the birthing center, and the 72-hour surgery hospital are probably the best answers to the question. The movement to provide posthospital care in less expensive extrahospital settings, such as nursing facilities, subacute postoperative recovery units, and physician office suites, is a portent of the transformations we face and the ongoing diffusion hospitals will likely suffer.

At some sort of virtual nexus, managed by what used to be the hospital executive group, may soon emerge the vital connection between all the different items on the growing menu of cost-effective alternative settings; from the traditional hospital unit to the subacute care facility to the patient's own bedroom.

HEALTH PLANS IN MOTION

Health plans enjoy the distinct marketplace advantage of scaleability. Product development, member services, and national accounts, which are the key aspects of the health plan business, are highly scaleable enterprises, and so plans can accumulate capital much more efficiently than doctors and hospitals, which have had such a hard time scaling their operations.

But all healthcare, like all politics, is local. How will the megaplans, like U.S. Healthcare/Aetna and the others, effectively transfer their best practices to every local practice and facility? They have to reinvent themselves every time they break into a new market. They cannot just transplant everything they know and do. They will still have to convince doctors and hospitals to convert to their systems. Doctors and hospitals might still be in business with lots of other health plans, so it is difficult to say who might have the leverage in some circumstances.

Is This Any Way to Run a Managed-Care Organization?

What is relatively easy to manage is the business risk in the risk pool, and health plans can do that as well as anyone. They can deliver protocols, practice guidelines, and standards and set up the reimbursement systems to push people in one direction. As long as there is excess supply, the plans can leverage member demand to gain advantage over a supply side that is hungry for business.

But is that managing care? For a health plan to get into the business of truly managing care, there has to be some kind of meaningful partnership with the caregivers. If health plans can earn a consonance in all the caregiver incentives they impose, then we might really have a shot at integrating care. It will not happen otherwise, or it might happen but independent of your health plan.

Doctors want to integrate care for all the right reasons, namely because it offers them a better way to care for their patients. Partner with physicians to change the incentives and they will eventually warm up to the idea. But most health plans today are not concerned about managing care. They are concerned about managing resources, and that is how they align the incentives. Only by incentivizing around managing care, improving health status, and enhancing outcomes will a plan forge a vital partnership with medical groups.

Talk to most physicians in managed-care lite and medium markets and you will find they do not like their health plans very much. It does not sound like much of a partnership, does it? You can never integrate care until you align the incentives, mission, and purpose of the health plan and the medical group. If payment systems are set at odds with physicians' interests, for example, or if the health plan dictates unacceptable conditions of care, the physicians can do little else but fight that payment system and those conditions of care at every turn.

Winning the Hearts and Minds of Physicians

If, on the other hand, the health plan recognizes that its future depends on how the physicians choose to practice, works hand-in-glove with doctors to stimulate better practices and freer information sharing, sets up the information technologies to facilitate sharing, establishes new incentives, and designs a supportive education system for members, a real partnership is born! There are tons and tons of similarly constructive actions a health plan can take to stimulate integration and true population health management. No matter how good your health plan, you can not make a rehab system or prevention program work without the eager cooperation of doctors.

The health plan business is wall-to-wall with speculators hustling to make a buck. At times the guiding principle of today's market seems to be, do whatever it takes. Physicians would gladly associate with a payor that shows it is concerned about moving toward integrated managed care, a system that better matches a doctor's practice preferences and ethics. What physicians want is a health plan that, while granting them freedom to practice medicine following their own best judgment, provides the information and opportunities to seriously discuss and, over time, establish best clinical practices. Physicians will not abide a plan that shoves them into ethical corners, where the right medical decision is not properly encouraged or even covered.

I say if your sole purpose is to make money and you have decided to accomplish that goal by managing resources, you will never be able to find the magic incentives for physicians to care for patients in any rational manner. Resource management, without a firm foundation in clinical management, is forever set at cross purposes against the responsible stewardship of population health.

Will insurance companies start funding groups to create their own provider arms? Not if they are smart. You cannot deliver managed care via a single product. Everyone, even Kaiser, is looking at alternatives to diversify. How can you either open up to other businesses or do something different within your existing network?

Again the managed-care pinwheel points the way toward a brighter future characterized by the free exchange of intellectual capital. Health plans need to accept their responsibility for achieving superior clinical outcomes by figuring out a way to work with a mass collection of data, starting to help providers emulate the best demonstrated practices, and measure clinical quality. A communitywide effort would be most effective. Rather than every HMO sending a questionnaire, so every medical group receives fifteen different ones, why not have the regional plans send a single questionnaire then share the results. Winning that kind of cooperation among competitors will take some doing!

What Spells Success

All in all, when HMOs or Independent Practice Associations (IPAs) compensate their primary-care physicians on a fee-for-service basis and capitate their specialists so they do not overutilize procedures, surgeries, and hospital beds, everybody wins. Consumers consistently list freedom of choice among their chief healthcare desires. With the right information technology and profiling, the right compensation and incentive system, and larger panels of more accessible specialists patients gain the freedom to choose. Payors and provider groups that follow this approach will take market share away from those who restrict doctors' and patients' freedom of choice.

Remember, our big problem today is hospital cost, not primary-care cost. Primary-care doctors drive but a small percentage of hospital days, so paying them discounted fee-for-service rates will not blow the budget. We have to look at the whole system. Some health plans argue that a gatekeeper model, in which the primary care physicians control the capitated pool for specialists, keeps costs down best. But patients just do not like it. Gatekeepers restrict freedom of choice. And every week we read in the newspaper about some other attack on managed care by consumer groups or litigating attorneys. The recent managed-care backlash in large part stems from the all-too-common perception that health plans too severely restrict choice and access.

It surprises some people to know that it is not always fancy in formation systems or sophisticated technologies a health plan needs to satisfy its members. More often I hear successful plans say, "We simply listened to our customers and responded to their complaints and suggestions." One health plan took the ingeniously simple step of installing a better phone system to make sure every single call was answered within two rings. Seniors especially can be impatient with phone communications. If you have to put a senior on hold and they do not hear music or some noise within about ten seconds, they are apt to think they got cut off and hang up. The little things mean a lot; ten seemingly trivial improvements add up to equal significantly higher customer satisfaction.

You do not even have to conduct patient satisfaction surveys when patients have freedom of choice. Let the marketplace work. Let primary-care physicians recommend specialists following their own best judgment, values, and customer choices. If we just set up a healthy competition between specialists to win referrals and build their panels, we will get better access to and efficiency from all specialists. Superior patient satisfaction will follow.

Somehow I fear, we have gotten away from letting the marketplace work in the traditional sense. With reengineered compensation methodologies and information technologies, there is no compelling reason not to reestablish natural market incentives.

PHYSICIAN GROUPS IN MOTION

Over the three years I spent in Great Britain as the head of a large healthcare consulting practice, one of the things the government did was change the incentives for general practitioners. They started out with just the right ratio: three general practitioners to every specialist. Then, almost as an afterthought, the reformers announced that any group practice serving more than 10,000 people would be granted a limited budget for which they would be tariffed.

The British effectively capitated their primary-care physicians and freed them to practice as they saw fit. One practitioner, operating a thriving stand-alone practice that served twice the national average number of patients per physician, raised eyebrows by referring clients to aroma therapists and all sorts of alternative providers. But by doing so he actually managed to eliminate all psychiatric consultations in his practice. It certainly was not his intended purpose for using alternative treatments, but it was an amazing consequence. He was managing care.

In America, many similar anecdotes enjoy wide circulation. Six internists, all of whom would surely make the top-ten list in their city, each served 1200 to 1500 seniors in addition to a strong commercial practice. Normally internists max out at 600 to 700 seniors each. Yet these doctors boasted the highest patient satisfaction rates and clinical quality measures. Asked the secret of their success, the physicians credited a deceptively simple mathematical model. For every 200 seniors added to the roster, the group hired one nurse practitioner to field questions and one extra person for telephone communication. Their telephone operators do not have computerized medical records, but they can call up detailed information regarding the patient's most recent visit. If a caller says he got a stomachache after taking his new pink pills, the nurse practitioner can render an on-the-spot remedy by advising him to reduce the dosage or take the pills after a meal.

Because the group's fully staffed phone support team can answer all inquiries so efficiently and keep in touch with seniors, many office visits are avoided without ever endangering anyone's health. And patients are more than happy to avoid the inconvenience and possibly the expense of an office visit. They just want the information they need to help themselves feel better. Of course a traditional fee-for-service group would be loath to employ the alternative caregivers or the telephones. That spells the difference between managing the operating budget and managing care.

Who Makes the Team?

Physicians will have to work more in teams to excel in the managed-care era. The successful individual players, whether in independent practice associations or group practices, will become superior at managing care by leading a team or understanding what it means to be a valuable, working part of a winning team.

The contemporary physician organization needs a management structure that puts one or two doctors in the top decision-making position. Such a structure is probably the most reliable indicator of how quickly a big medical group or IPA can respond to marketplace changes. A democratic arrangement, in which every doctor gets a vote on every decision, will slow the group to a crawl.

Alternative treatments and caregivers, such as nurse practitioners or chiropractors, might be integral parts of the new team concept. The AMA can object to the very thought of nursing professionals rendering primary care, but every signpost points the responsible managed-care organization in that direction. The managed-care practitioner's only concern, after all, should be for the health of a membership.

In selecting their managed-care partners, seasoned physician group executives tell me they are very careful about with whom they tie up. Get your toe wet first, they say. Learn a bit about the plan, but do not be unduly influenced by it. Make yourself a better, smarter business partner but remain true to your ideals. Running the kind of practice you want will attract the kind of patients you want.

Look at the board. What is its purpose? What do board members talk about? Are they solely concerned about price earning ratios, payoff to shareholders, and other financial results? Do they ever talk about healthcare itself? Are they worried about what might happen to plan members? How does the board deal with the ethical problems of coverage? Does it phase healthcare coverage?

Compared to most physician-run entities, managed-care organizations are run by superior business talents. The chief danger is getting caught up in the business side and losing sight of your values and principles as a physician. Too many physicians today are vulnerable, scared, and grabbing at straws. They wonder, will patients come. In resolving these fears and wonders, even the most sophisticated medical groups will be hard pressed to outwit the managed-care companies.

Too many physicians have rushed into IPA formation on the baseless advice that they can coast along, make an independent public offering, and walk away with a bushel of cash. This is ridiculous. A few may somehow succeed but most will surely fail.

The Carrot on a Stick

There is no such thing as a neutral incentive, in managed care or anywhere, but physician incentives can and should be effectively neutralized in terms of resource consumption and costs. A plan should not pay physicians more or less depending on what they do for a patient; it should pay them more or less based on how effectively they care for populations under their responsibility, against agreed-upon standards, and it should pay them more or less depending on how effectively they are responding to the needs and desires and requirements of the membership.

The prevalent notion that plans should link physicians' resource use to payment is sadly misguided. Fee-for-service, discounted fee-for-service, withholds, and gatekeepers, those are methods for managing resources, not care. Resources are merely one vehicle by which you achieve the best possible outcomes, sometimes the better outcome takes more and sometimes fewer resources.

The standard approach is to develop protocols and then, through incentive and care review systems, to impose those protocols on practitioners. Here is where the war breaks out. The very notion of exploiting physician oversupply and leveraging the situation to reduce resource utilization and variation is a declaration of war between the health plan and its medical staff. That is no synergistic partnership, it is probably not a sustainable business relationship, and it is certainly a poor strategy for quality patient care.

Instead, when risk managers instead engage physicians in a dialogue based on accurate information, they can much more effectively change behaviors and achieve better practices. The managed-care organizations that can do this best, one might argue, are going to be the sure winners. They will say, "Here is our utilization management review process. Hammer it out with your colleagues, and if you have any questions or suggestions, we are ready to talk." This tactic offers an equally effective and far more professional approach to controlling hospital utilization and practice patterns.

The Accountability Thing

All professionals today have to get used to being held accountable for their actions, that is accountable to their peers, to their patients, to a university, or to society at large. A strong chain of accountability enables health plans to manage as close as possible to the point of service. Those who render a service know best how it should be managed, so the plan must give medical professionals more flexibility by properly communicating and aligning their accountabilities.

I hear it over and over again that medical staffs have only themselves to blame for their weak position in the current managed-care marketplace. They put themselves in this spot. They paid lip service to collective responsibility, accountability, and self-discipline but they never did anything about it. So what happened? State governments in the past few years have slapped physicians down, wrestled control away from them, and put lawyers in charge of them. The medical staff that behaves responsibly and is clearly perceived to be providing quality services to its population is still going to be treated with respect.

Medical groups, too, need to adopt an epidemiologic approach and reinvent themselves to embrace the health risks associated with defined populations. The people who run health plans are growing weary of fighting with medical staffs. Some physicians could organize and feed their hunger for control. The potential weakness of physician-run managed care plans is their propensity to grow too big for their defined populations.

Brave New Physician Groups

Physician-run organizations will drive change, not only on the physician side but across the full continuum of care delivery and across the managed-care pinwheel. Large groups will continue to expand, and some will do their best to break into the HMO business. The lasting success of such ventures is questionable, at best. Once again it is a matter of physicians acquiring the size, scale, and capital needed to operate a viable insurance enterprise.

This is not to say that physician groups will not be formidable managed-care organizations in their own right. Today's major groups are designed to incorporate group models, group practices, independent physicians through IPA models, and some physicians in MSO-type models who still own their practices but are managed by an outside managed-care organization. In any market such a large and complex group bothers to enter, they normally strive to be number one or number two with a 20 or 30% market share. A group could maybe get by on a strong reputation and access, but in the end it will have to size up and deliver. As markets evolve, many will see three or four major players, with a similar variety of group structures, move to the front of the pack. And in California, we are starting to see that already. Sacramento, for instance, has shaken down to four players: Kaiser, Mercy System, Sutter System, and Foundation.

Physicians do not really want to be in the insurance business, they do not want to be an HMO, and they do not want to be a hospital. There has to be some balance in the system. Physicians know they do not have the insurance underwriting expertise. But lately they have accumulated plenty of contracting, medical management, and delivery expertise.

Make no mistake, physicians watch the healthcare market with a sharp eye. A lot of HMOs are wondering how they can move into the indemnity side or the PPO side, because they need to offer that triple option to attract employers. So from the physician group perspective, a development such as the U.S. Healthcare-Aetna merger makes perfect sense. Now physicians are waiting to see whether the plan can pull off its broader strategy and decide what to do with all the group business Aetna had just nicely started to create.

Medical groups are busy consolidating on the bankrupt theory that the only way to recoup profitability is to grow big enough to act as the insurance company and take the HMOs right out of the picture. Big mistake. We need to return to the notion of partnership between a network of entities, each occupying a protective niche in which they excel. The successful insurance company will be the one that cultivates win/win partnerships with provider entities, such as partnerships that fall short of ownership. Likewise, the successful provider entity will be the one that joins in such partnerships with insurance companies, again falling short of actually owning the insurance business. HMOs are selling their staff models as fast they possibly can, because it finally dawned on them that they lack the physician expertise. You can already see those pinwheels spinning.

The Primary Care Base

A solid primary-care physician group will enjoy many opportunities in tomorrow's managed-care market. But even the most successful stand-alone family practices are going to have a hard time getting the capital and information they will need to survive and thrive on the managed-care pinwheel. The undeniable attraction of today's larger groups is that they can easily provide a single point for contracting and member access. Participating primary-care physician organizations may still retain some local autonomy, while gaining invaluable access to vital capital and information. One simply cannot run a family practice these days without participating in community-health management by building strong working relations with health plans, other physicians, and hospital systems.

In moving from managed-care lite to heavy, primary-care physicians will face a greater and greater need for infrastructure and information. Doctors are not just seeing patients in the office anymore. A practice needs a structure to manage more risk, to manage those costs on the institutional side, to manage the contracting issues, and to deliver all the information physicians need to drive the overall medical care process.

What every self-respecting primary-care group should be asking itself is, How do we manage the medical process better? Like all other managed-care provider entities, physician groups should distinguish themselves by concentrating always on the medical side rather than the financial side. Yes, all physicians would like to secure better contracts and better reimbursement. Growing market pressure is bound to spoil some of the fun, as one group executive puts it. So every primary-care group must start to think seriously about how they are going to achieve superior quality outcomes in the most cost-effective manner.

More and more primary-care doctors are practicing in multispecialty groups. As they watch their specialist colleagues' reimbursement rates freefall, some will be tempted to force radical adjustments in relative compensation levels. Such an extremely divisive gesture may paralyze groups from being able to really pursue the quality initiatives, the contracting initiatives with payors, and the training initiatives everyone wants physicians to pursue; if every meeting focuses on compensation, no one will have the time to get any worthwhile business done.

Soon the tables may turn, and primary-care physicians may come to invite specialists to organize with them, but at arm's length.

What is So Special About Specialists?

In a fascinating development, specialists are aggregating along single-specialty lines and bidding for managed-care contracts. Some might call it a further fragmentation of care, but many feel that specialty contracting will more probably facilitate a rational focusing around core technologies and a breakdown of core medical processes into more reasonably manageable bits.

Again, though, doctors surely do not need to become insurers to be winners in the managed care future. What the aspiring specialist groups really need are management service organizations (MSOs). Tailored to meet a group's extraclinical management needs, an MSO offers comprehensive services that usually include very sophisticated information technology and systems administration, contract negotiation, quality outcome analysis, and data severity adjustment. Saving hospital days is the MSO's chief reason for existence.

In managed-care heavy markets, payors might soon be encouraging discounted fee-for-service for primary-care physicians and capitation of specialists. Eventually, the right model might pay specialists based on the size of their panels, not on the procedures billings or procedure-based point systems that some health plans have concocted. Specialist panels have to be severity-adjusted, too, so the better specialists who attract tougher cases are appropriately remunerated for their vital role.

Finally, a bit of friendly advice to specialists. Organize into a network broad enough that you can either build or lease a very sophisticated information system and hire some enlightened and highly experienced managed-care executives. The contemporary specialty group's main goal should be to develop products that convincingly demonstrate measurably lower utilization with improved quality.

PHARMACEUTICAL HOUSES IN MOTION

The big drug companies have been orchestrating a major advance into the managed-care realm. Several pharmacy benefits management firms, wholly owned or operated by drug manufacturers, have already taken the lead in areas such as outcomes research, clinical protocol development, and disease management.

There is a synergy between pharmacy benefit management and physician management. Physicians write all those prescriptions, and if we start to funnel better clinical information directly to physicians, in real time via the electronic medical record concept, physicians will change their practice patterns based on what they learn. Vast numbers may start prescribing the more effective drug, even though it has the higher price. They may stop using generics. The more expensive drug, many will see, may facilitate the best clinical outcome, which is usually the best economic result, too. Once we start to understand how we can manage the outcomes and the medical process, versus just managing costs, we may see a whole different pattern of behavior and care emerge.

The drug companies have finally gotten back to basics. In the fee-for-service world, pharmaceutical manufacturers just marketed their most expensive products. Today's customers select drugs not just based on the acquisition cost but also considering the total long-term economic impact of using that drug in a clinically sound regimen. The major pharmaceutical manufacturers, at the vanguard of the exciting new outcomes research field, are moving swiftly to fund groundbreaking studies that can prove how the utilization of expensive but more cost-effective drugs can reap lower overall healthcare costs.

With an important educational role to fill, strong economic muscles to flex, and an invaluable research and development function to perform, the pharmaceutical houses promise to be faithful partners in many aspects of the managed-care mission. Virtually every other sector of the industry, payor, provider, physician, and member alike will benefit from drug manufacturers' increased sharing of vital intellectual capital.

AGAINST AESTHETES AND ANARCHISTS

Yes, managed care is a serious game that takes just minutes to learn but a lifetime to master. Some say we can speed things along by modifying present systems, keeping the best of the old and incorporating the most promising of the new. Others say we would do better to rip everything down and start over from scratch.

Both are wrong, both are right. Our healthcare system is due for a complete overhaul but the transition must be orderly and stepwise. When naval architects rebuild a sailing ship, though every board, every nail, every seam of caulk might be replaced, the ship nevertheless retains its original name. So it will be as we rebuild our healthcare system.

Sound Industrial Redesign

We have reengineered an awful lot of processes, merged and acquired at such a pace that you need a program to keep the names straight, sent hordes of dedicated employees packing, and purchased and installed the latest technologies and somehow without really changing the ways we do business. For all this progress we have a prominent school of healthcare aesthetes to thank. They have busied themselves changing all the design elements that do not really matter, that do not really add value to our healthcare system, and that do not really figure into the health of our communities.

What the healthcare world needs now is not impressive aesthetic design but solid industrial design, in the purest sense of that misunderstood discipline. Henry Petroski, one of America's top engineering minds, carefully distinguishes merely aesthetic problems from true industrial design problems. His most keenly illustrative example concerns another game that takes just minutes to learn but a lifetime to master, chess.

Unlike, a can opener, a chess set offers few if any prospects for the earnest industrial designer. The layout of the board and the number and distinct functions of the pieces having been fixed long ago, the design of a "new" chess set is a strictly aesthetic problem. "And in the name of aesthetics," Petroski complains, "Many a chess set has been made more modern- or abstract-looking, if not merely different-looking, at the expense of chess players' ability to tell the queen from the king or the knight from the bishop."[*]

---

[*]Petroski, Henry *The Evolution of Useful Things* (New York: Vintage Books, 1994) pp. 32–33.

Much of the industrial design activity in the early days of managed care has hovered at this aesthetic level. Soon we will get around to reinventing the game, its overall object, the number and distinct functions of the pieces, and the very way the outcome is contested. We will be calling on the complete industrial designers, who are concerned with how our healthcare system "will behave at the hands of its intended, and perhaps unintended, users." Healthcare's true industrial designers will find little glamour and no glory in their chosen field. Petroski, whose core thesis is that form follows *failure,* not function, characterizes the industrial designer's predicament as follows:

> The individual designer and engineer involved in the creation of large systems is often lost in numerous management shuffles, and the story of the end product is frequently that of a major production with an anonymous if professional cast of thousands, no single one of whom is commonly known to be the designer or the engineer. (*The Evolution of Useful Things,* pp. 78-79)

He might as well be describing the healthcare industry today. Healthcare's most valuable industrial designers will be judged not by their elegant engineering solutions or grand architectural feats but by their capacity to learn a certain humility, to right what they know, and to stick around maybe just long enough to make sure a core process or two gets properly redesigned from the ground up. All lasting change is made of such humble contributions.

Power to the People

Healthcare consumers want more choice, and they are getting it in today's competitive market. The number of health insurers offering a point-of-service alternative nearly doubled over the past five years.*

The objective and the effect have been to woo people out of traditional indemnity coverage and into managed-care plans.

The question is: Can a person with a point-of-service option really be a health plan member in good standing? A member with any serious illness could hardly afford the penalty of going out of network for sophisticated and expensive diagnoses, treatments, therapies, and drugs. A pro-

---

*Hagland, Mark, "Point-of-service: Staying alive," *Hospitals & Health Networks,* 20 October 1996, p. 58.

longed hospitalization can easily bankrupt a family if the member has to foot much of the bill. For many, the offer of more choice for your premium dollar will amount to a clever illusion. But it might just succeed in enrolling a host of previously reluctant populations, especially Medicare recipients.

More than an option for greater choice, offered up by health plans like it is some kind of gift, members should demand the information they need to make intelligent decisions about their own health. This information age we live in will provide the means for robust, a communications infrastructure by which a health plan can inform and educate its membership as well as market to the community at large. Already the consumer health information available on World Wide Web pages is doing a world of good.

Here in my own backyard, Long Beach Community Medical Center operates a 200-page Web site offering basic medical science information, other educational materials, and interactive capabilities. The site gets some 700 hits a day and, according to the program managers, has been a wild success in encouraging and aiding patients to play a vital role in their own health and healthcare.*

Our managed-care future will be built upon such innovative uses of technology to disseminate information and communicate with populations at risk. But the information and the responsibility of managing it cannot reside with a health plan, a hospital system, or a physician practice alone. These communitywide interactive programs, such as must be situated at the very hub of the managed-care pinwheel.

MANAGED HEALTHCARE AND THE ACADEMICS

Shortly after having planted the germ of this book, I published an open letter to our nation's medical academics. That letter** is still freshness dated for today's managed care market.

Legislative reform (the letter began) was a snooze as a mystery thriller—sleuths with too many clues, suspects with too many motives, the action choked by too many convoluted subplots. Now here I go spoiling the ending.

---

*Hagland, Mark, "Power to the Patient," *Hospitals & Health Networks,* 20 October 1996, p. 28-30.
**Patterson, Dennis J., "Managed care: Far from academic," *Hospitals & Health Networks,* Last Word, 5 May 1995, p. 74.

Astute readers and viewers have known it all along: tomorrow's healthcare marketplace will be driven by a renewed zeal for efficiency and value and will feature integrated financing and delivery systems that manage care for large populations. The American business community has been enacting such reforms for over a decade, and those with the firmest grip on our healthcare future have been devoted students of managed care, not *Congressional Record* subscribers or C-SPAN addicts.

No one more urgently needs a crash course on managed care than do the trustees of our nation's medical universities. Good trusteeship today requires a rather intricate knowledge of managed-care concepts, practices, and trends. Lacking proper leadership, the very teaching and research core of our healthcare system could be in danger. The impending revolution is bound to hit campus like a student uprising.

Universities Face Unique Challenges

Today's medical academic centers includes a troublesome variety of entities, such as a hospital, a faculty practice plan, ambulatory care facilities, and in some cases, a health maintenance organization. Often, teaching facilities are located in declining urban neighborhoods and serve more than their fair share of Medicaid recipients and the uninsured. Meanwhile, traditional sources of revenue are drying up as the market braces for stiffer competition, prepares for legislative reforms, and gropes for equitable solutions to the medical liability problem. Managing business risk is difficult enough for any healthcare organization these days and for the academic medical center it is doubly challenging.

Managed care poses timely answers for the academics, if only governors would answer the challenge. Aiming to keep its members healthy and satisfied, a managed-care organization creates appropriate business incentives for payors and providers alike, keeps costs down without sacrificing quality by providing the right care in the right setting, and champions the fundamental doctor-patient relationship.

The population enrolled in managed-care health plans grows every day. More and more employers are restricting or repackaging benefits to encourage employees to join managed-care plans. Governments, too, are moving large populations into managed care by allowing HMOs to enroll Medicare and Medicaid recipients. And why not? The government gets a discount on premiums, HMOs and providers boost their volumes, and Medicare and Medicaid members enjoy first-class service, something our Veterans Administration hospital system really ought to consider.

Most still think of their managed-care volume as extra business, but it is really converted indemnity business, recaptured at about 50 cents on the dollar. We must reinvent the academic medical center to compete at that revenue level. All but the very most sophisticated and specialized services provided at university hospitals are now commonly available for better prices at other community facilities. University hospitals and faculty have been at odds and managed care demands their cooperation. Specialists now dominate the faculty and managed care demands a strong primary-care network and a corresponding shift in power. University institutions usually charge the highest prices in town for superior quality but high quality at high prices just will not cut it in the managed-care era.

Change Begins with the Trustee

Is your institution managed-care friendly? Ask yourself the following:

- How much of our current business is with managed-care organizations, and is that proportion growing as it should be?
- Do we have a strong primary care network that will allow our institutions to take on capitated payments and cover lives for HMOs that wish to contract with us?
- How do our costs compare to our current managed-care fee-for-service discounts or per diems?
- Have we appointed an executive to prepare our medical and clinical staffs for capitation?
- Have we incorporated our answers to these questions into our strategic plan and gauged the impact on our future needs for beds, outpatient services, skilled nursing facilities, and home health care?

Ultimately, teaching medicine and delivering care are distinct roles. The managed-care academic would do well to create a corporate entity, unencumbered by the university's slow decision processes, that can quickly network, sign contracts, merge, and integrate. The partition between the two should be high enough that, if the business entity fails, university resources will be protected.

In days ahead, our university communities will be seeking our critical guidance. Let us tell the real-life drama: the chase scene was fun, but the climax could be a bloody shoot-out. Please resist the instinctive urge to avert your eyes.

STILL MORE BELLWETHERS

Webster's Collegiate Dictionary, 10th ed. defines a bellwether as the sheep that leads a flock, an indicator of trends. Despite the connotation of a herd mentality, bellwethers provide those wonderful intangibilities without which the ambitious prognosticator would soon be at a complete loss for words. More loosely, I say bellwethers are the things that make me stop and say, "Gee, all the data show and all the pundits say things are going the other way, but in my gut I feel this trend deserves a closer look."

In my travels I have collected pithy managed-care bellwethers like some people collect charms or refrigerator magnets. Assembled here are several gut feelings and words of advice that found no better place in our discourse, but demand consideration none the less.

- Put your money on new players. Upstart entrepreneurs, with a fresh outlook and no stubborn traditions to break, will bring more flexibility and quicker decision making to the alternative and postacute care markets.
- Healthcare's big buyers will be the trendsetters; the smaller buyers and brokers will just get sucked up in the whirlwind and plopped back down on the hard ground.
- Managed care eventually comes down to customer satisfaction and understanding, and more than any drastic action or fancy deals, that will require excellent communication and market research.
- Look for companies that are grabbing more market share, then find out why!
- A sufficiently organized consumer backlash against managed care, such as a powerful consumer lobby, or special interest group, or regulatory structure could freeze the unprepared or poorly performing managed-care organization right in its tracks.
- Major purchasing coalitions and government entities are getting ever more sophisticated about what is happening inside the managed-care organizations and how they manage risk pools, and they are beginning to think in terms of adjusting risk and establishing appropriate measures of clinical outcomes.

- Perhaps we will move away from payor-managed care and toward care managed by healthcare professionals, which could be a real boon for the academic medical centers, who would become the absolute dictators of care standards.

- Hospitals realize they are in the middle of managed care when medical groups start complaining, "You are not helping us manage bed days very well, and if you do not wise up we are going to redirect our patients elsewhere." It takes just a tiny amount of lost business to get a hospital's undivided attention. On the flip side, a physician group could lose 25 or 30 percent of its practice before the message sinks in that, "Hey, guys! We are in this managed-care world for the duration."

Another bellwether commonly sighted on the horizon is some new way of paying health plans based on risk pools and on how well different organizations care for very sick patients. Massachusetts, for example, has been experimenting with how it pays health plans, which they suspect are lagging behind indemnity insurers in terms of the quality of care they provide and the levels of risk they accept. The state wants to pay plans based on risk-adjusted data that reflect actual clinical outcomes.

A sudden insistence on demonstrated value could throw a wrench in the whole managed-care movement, because so many so-called managed-care plans still reap the bulk of their efficiency by managing resources and risk. Many may not be equal to the challenge of actually managing care and health. But is true health management not the bellwether we all should be following into the future? It is easier to say than it will be to do.

S U M M A R Y

The time to contemplate managed care's best- and worst-case scenarios is now, as our adventure is only just beginning.

Best case is the wholly integrated delivery system and total population health management squiggling like mirages on the distant horizon. To make the vision real and ensure their safe arrival in Boomtown, many aspiring pioneers prepare for a hard ride over rough country. The managed-care terrain grows more hospitable, slowly but surely, with each leg of the long journey.

Worst case is too casually surveyed and hastily constructed, our shiny new integrated delivery systems and virtual networks become so many ghost towns, built by an overpromoted dream on an overexploited landscape. Will even a signboard remain standing to remind future generations of our grand folly?

It is rare that somebody comes along and completely redefines the game. The seeds of prepaid practice were sown way back in the 1950s, and more power to those astute enough to have watched and learned from the cooperative movement in the northern United States, Canada, and other such pioneering efforts. Right now, buffeted by chaos and uncertainty and the perceived avarice and bad decisions of profiteering HMOs, our healthcare system is swinging on a tightrope. At times it seems the whole system might plummet to certain extinction or swing back to an arrangement more akin to a fee-for-service, professionally dominated environment.

Let me conclude this chapter and this section by saying again what most certainly bears repeating here: Only the free exchange of intellectual capital through advanced information technology and case management techniques, all with a sharp eye toward better health outcomes, will keep managed care moving in the right direction. We have arrived at one of those defining moments in history, when we enjoy some luxury of choice, the strong guidance of wisdom, and real hope for a better future. What will we make of the opportunity? Our managed-care trajectory will send us soaring and, thanks to responsive controls and skillful piloting, will see the healthcare industry safely back where it belongs: serving the people who so depend on it.

5
CHAPTER

The Managed-Care Index—Your Marketplace At-a-Glance

Successful healthcare strategists have long been aware that there is no acceptable substitute for a deep knowledge of one's own local service area, population, and market players. Such knowledge never comes easy, though. To forge a dynamic tool and cultivate a living discipline for establishing such a knowledge base, today's planners must embrace *managed care* as an umbrella term that encompasses all the participants and component forces in a changing marketplace, as were introduced in Chapters 3 and 4. These forces can be quantified, meaningfully compared to historical and national data, weighed, and aggregated by applying the new disciplines and techniques of managed-care indexing.

The managed-care index promises to be a highly useful tool for measuring the level of managed-care presence, and something of the pace and momentum of change, in any market. In this two-chapter section of *Indexing Managed Care* you will learn how to construct a vivid model of your organization's future marketplace. This chapter presents the chief components of the managed-care index and establishes its conceptual framework, its basic construction, key indicators of managed-care presence, and milestones along the journey from a managed-care lite to a managed-care heavy market. The next chapter considers reliable sources of fresh data, explains how those data are input, and walks you through the various calculations for index scoring.

DAWN OF THE INDEX

Dr. Ian Morrison and I, assisted by his colleagues at the Institute for the Future, created the managed-care index in 1993. What we wanted was an accurate, meaningful, objective, and understandable measure of the actual presence of managed care across the nation or in any local marketplace. The tool we envisioned would be built upon widely available data but would imaginatively digest those data, subject them to rigorous analysis, churn them into useable information, and finally report managed-care's progress as a simple percentage, that is, one hard number between zero and one hundred, with zero percent indicating an all fee-for-service market and one hundred percent indicating a fully managed-care market.

We figured that by getting some idea of how payors, physicians, and hospitals were trying to wield control over each other and over the health-care community at large, we could track any market's evolution from managed-care lite to managed-care heavy. So we assembled an expert panel, including the dean of a medical school, the head of the National Coalition on Quality Assurance, and the Health Care Financing Administration's top actuary, and asked them what they thought about our indicators and weights. Based on their enthusiastic responses and sound advice, we refined the index and, using proxy data, calculated managed-care presence at about 20.44% nationwide in 1993.

That calculated level of managed care presence fit nicely with Dr. Morrison's and my gut feelings about the state of managed care in the United States in 1993 and, so, confirmed that our method and our metrics were on the right track. At this point, our indexing tool was all but ready for other strategic planners to customize and use to measure managed care presence in their own local markets.

CONSTRUCTION OF THE INDEX

I anticipate that different readers will be studying and using this index in varying degrees of depth. Those most keenly interested in the science of the index will want to turn to Appendix B, which presents the actual weightings and the 1993 baselines set by an expert panel at the Institute for the Future. But for those of us who are less statistically inclined and more practitioners or students of managed care, I have devised a friendlier and easier-to-use indexing tool.

Constructed of simple pie charts, this indexing method invites you to apply your expert knowledge to roughly illustrate how extensively each sector of your market uses the various managed-care techniques by which the index gauges managed-care presence. The text provides instructions for assembling and shading in pie slices, each representing a certain aspect of the technique and each sized according to the index weight of that aspect.

Once assembled from these shaded slices, the whole pie will show how much your market employs that technique. The completed pies should give you a visual feel for where your market is today and, more important, give you a basis for future planning.

Use your own knowledge of your own market, available data, and better judgment in hazarding what we call Scientific Wild Assuming Guess (SWAG). First shade in the slices to indicate how the technique is being used at present. As a further exercise, you may want to predict where your market will be in five years. Extra pie workcharts are provided in Appendix A.

In most cases the first question about the technique is not recorded on the pie chart; it is shown to give the reader a feel for the lite end of the continuum. After each first question we show the whole pie chart and then break down the components for ease of completion. At the end of each section we include our "Expert Panel" estimates, as calculated by The Institute of the Future in 1993.

USERS

The users sector is divided into two main components: (1) patient managed-care incentives and (2) enrollee provider panel restrictions.

Patient Managed-Care Incentives

This indicator concerns the incentives (and disincentives) that influence the behavior of patients and enrollees. The index categorizes patient managed-care incentives along the following scales. For each scale shade the chart accordingly.

Patient Managed-Care Incentives

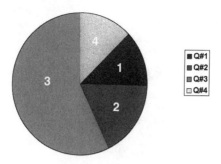

Q#1   No health insurance: leave slice blank for % uninsured

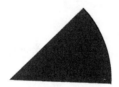

Q#2   Insurance combinations of copayment

■ Insured with deductible under $100: blacken ⅓ of slice
■ Insured with deductible/copayment $100-$200
■ Insured with deductible/copayment above $200: blacken entire slice

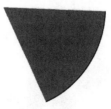

Q#3   Financial incentives

■ No financial incentives: leave pie slice blank
■ Financial incentive to use restricted panels (1%-10%)

- Financial incentive to use restricted panels (10%-29%)
- Financial incentive to use restricted panels (30%-99%): blacken entire slice

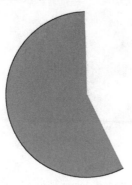

Q#4   Panel restrictions

- No restrictions: leave pie slice blank
- Restricted panel for primary care
- Restricted panel for all medical care
- Restricted panel for all healthcare (mental health, drug abuse, optometrist, diagnostic test, pharmaceuticals): blacken entire slice

In 1993, using its best SWAG, The Institute for the Future shaded the patient managed-care incentives pie as follows:

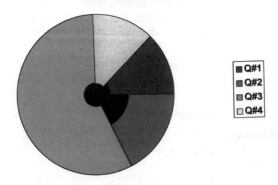

Enrollee Provider Panel Restrictions

This indicator concerns the incentives (and disincentives) that influence patients' and enrollees' choice of physicians. The index categorizes patient managed-care incentives along the following six factors. Please shade each slice to show the percentage of the enrollee population you believe has the following payor restrictions on choice of physician.

Enrollee Provider Panel Restrictions

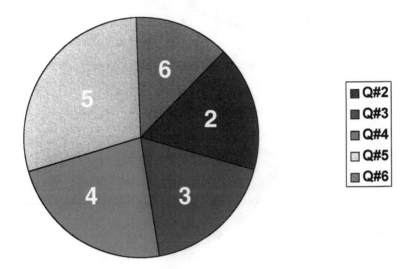

- ■ Q#2
- ■ Q#3
- ▣ Q#4
- ▢ Q#5
- ▨ Q#6

Q#1   No restrictions: do not record

Q#2   Network, 10% or less copayment to go outside:

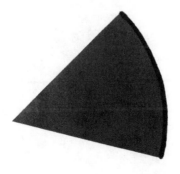

Q#3   Network, 11% or more copayment to go outside:

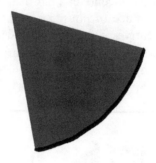

Q#4   Network with gatekeeper, up to 29% or more copayment:

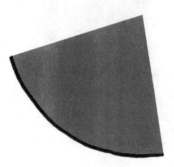

Q#5   Network with gatekeeper, 30% or more copayment:

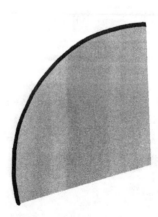

Q#6   Closed panel without point-of-service:

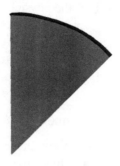

In 1993, The Institute for the Future made the following baseline estimates for enrollee provider panel restrictions.

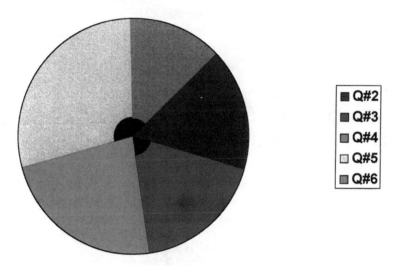

PROVIDERS

The providers sector is divided into two main components: (1) physician providers and (2) hospital providers.

Physician Providers

The index gives significant weighting to the physician practice component, as hospital executives should note when crafting a strategic plan. The provider side of the index is weighted 77.2% in favor of the physicians and only 22.8% for hospitals. The hospitals have the resources in terms of money and space, but under managed care the physicians are in the driver's seat.

The index considers five physician provider techniques: (1) process management of pharmaceuticals, (2) physician financial structures, (3) medical process management of physicians, (4) organizational structure of physician practice setting, and (5) physician referral access.

Process Management of Pharmaceuticals

This indicator concerns the restrictions placed on the physicians by the payors or contracting body. Again, blacken each pie slice for the amount of a physician's practice that you believe or know have these restrictions in their contract.

Q#1   No restrictions on prescribing: do not record

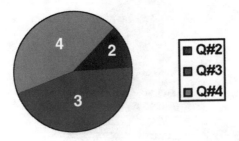

Q#2   No review or restricted formulary—shade % of pie slice that has some restrictions

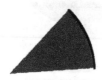

Q#3   Pharmacist review and formulary

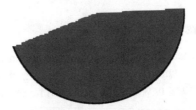

Q#4   Medical director review and use of formulary

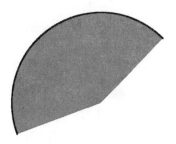

In 1993, The Institute for the Future estimated the use of the process management of pharmaceuticals technique as follows:

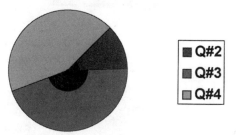

Physician Financial Structures

This indicator concerns the financial incentives (and disincentives) that influence the behavior of physicians. The index categorizes physician financial structures along the following scales. Please shade each slice to indicate the proportion of physician practices you believe are receiving the following incentives for the entire populations they serve.

Q#1   Unmanaged fee-for-service: do not record

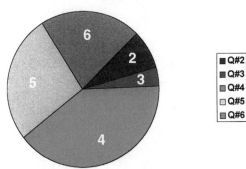

Q#2   Discounted fee-for-service

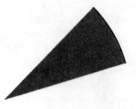

Q#3   Fee-for-service with risk pools

Q#4   Primary care physicians are capitated

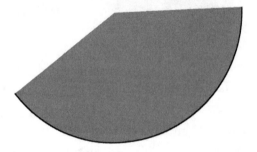

Q#5 Specialists are capitated

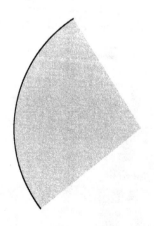

Q#6   Global capitation

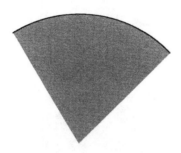

In 1993, The Institute for the Future estimated the use of the physician financial structures technique as follows:

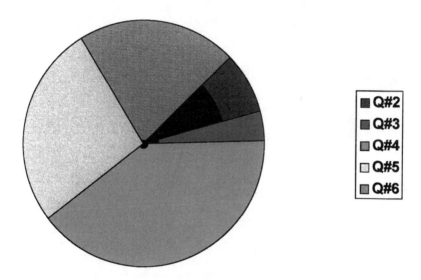

Medical Process Management of Physicians

This indicator concerns the medical micromanagement of physicians using various utilization review and cultural controls. The index categorizes medical process management whether or not it is imposed by the payor, an Independent Practice Association (IPA), or any other entity, such as a Management Service Organization (MSO). You know the drill. Shade each slice to show the proportion of physician practices that uses the following techniques for the entire populations they serve.

Q#1   No review: do not record

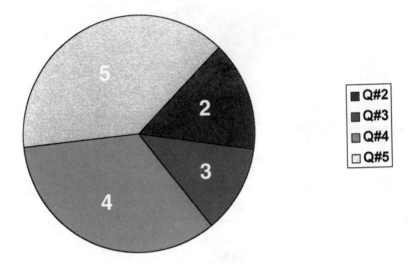

Q#2   Light utilization review (retroactive review)

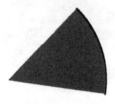

Q#3   Light process management (prior authorization)

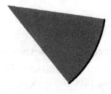

Q#4   Heavy process management (prior and concurrent reviews)

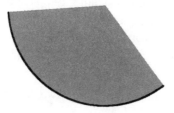

Q#5   Cultural controls (including heavy process management)

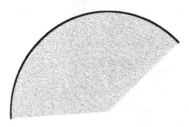

In 1993, The Institute for the Future estimated the use of a medical process management of physicians technique as follows:

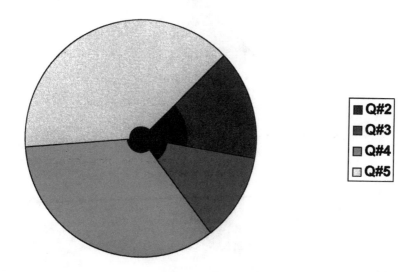

Organizational Structure of Physician Practice Setting

This indicator concerns the physician group size and level of integration. The index categorizes the organization structure of physician practice settings on a scale from solo practioner to integrated medical system. Shade each slice to show the percentage of physicians practicing under these arrangements in your marketplace.

Q#1   Independent practice, one or two doctors: do not record

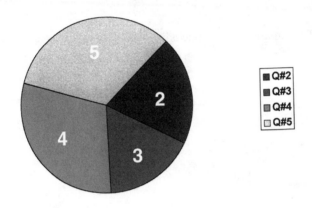

Q#2   Single-specialty group or IPA practice

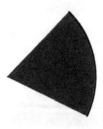

Q#3   Small multispecialty group or IPA practice

Q#4   Medium multispecialty group or IPA practice

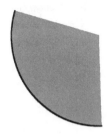

Q#5   Large multispecialty group

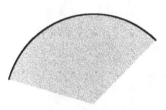

In 1993, The Institute for the Future estimated the organizational structure of physician practice setting as follows:

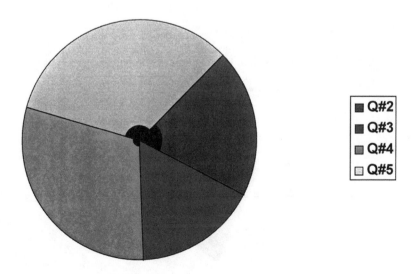

Physician Referral Access

This indicator concerns the restrictions placed on physicians to refer patients and enrollees to other physicians. The index categorizes physician referral access based on insurance type and panels. Shade each slice to show the access controls on physician practices for the entire populations they serve.

Q#1   No restrictions: do not record

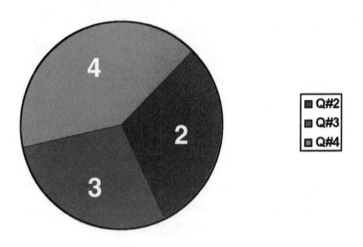

Q#2   Preferred Provider Organization (PPO) (general restrictions)

Q#3   Closed panel restrictions (some specialties)

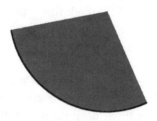

Q#4   Closed panel restrictions (all specialties)

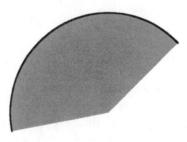

In 1993, The Institute for the Future estimated the restriction of physician referral access as follows:

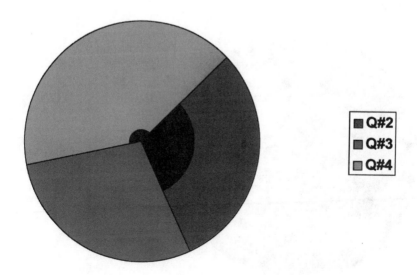

Hospital Providers

For managed-care techniques used by hospitals, the managed-care index allocates a weight of 22.8%. Although this represents the minority share of the providers portion of the index, it reflects that hospitals today are really dealing with a multitude of strategies, only one of which is managed care. We discuss the implications of this fact later in the book. For integrated delivery systems, especially, it will be important to understand the impact of all hospital strategies across the entire pinwheel.

The index considers three hospital provider techniques: (1) Medicare risk contracting, (2) hospital medical-process management, and (3) risk sharing among hospitals, physicians, and payors.

Medicare Risk Contracting Percentage

This indicator concerns the penetration of managed care into a market's Medicare population. The index scale for Medicare risk contracting, figured on a strict percentage basis using Health Care Financing Administration (HCFA) data, will surely evolve as the federal government moves more and more of the Medicare population into managed-care products. The index scale is a simple percentage of the Medicare eligible population that is enrolled in managed-care risk products.

Medicare Risk

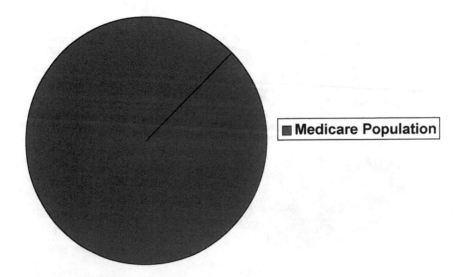

Medicare Population

In 1993, Medicare risk contracting was estimated to cover 7% of the eligible population. The figure has grown significantly since then.

Medicare Population

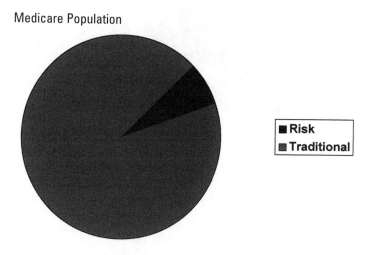

■ Risk
■ Traditional

Hospital Medical Process Management

This indicator concerns the sophistication hospitals exhibit in micromanaging core medical processes for optimum efficiency and effectiveness. The index categorizes hospital medical process management along six criteria. Go ahead, shade each pie slice to indicate the percentage of patients who have these techniques used on them during a hospital stay in your community.

Q#1   No restrictions: do not record

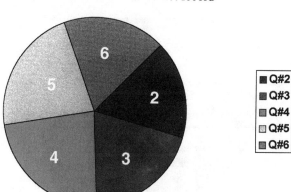

■ Q#2
■ Q#3
■ Q#4
■ Q#5
■ Q#6

Q#2   Preadmission certification (only)

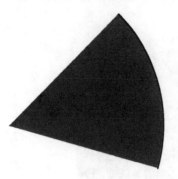

Q#3   Discharge planning

Q#4   Concurrent utilization review (case management)

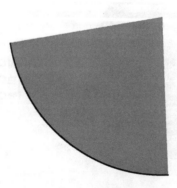

Q#5   Detailed practice guidelines or critical pathways

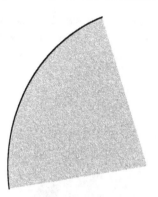

Q#6   Clinical continuous quality improvement/total quality management

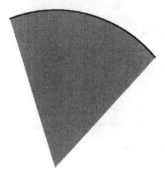

In 1993, The Institute for the Future estimated the use of hospital medical-process management as follows:

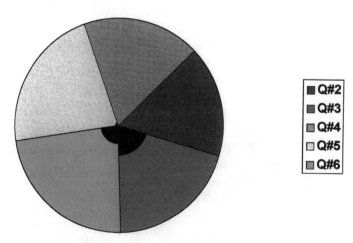

Risk Sharing Among Hospitals, Physicians, and Payors

This indicator concerns the extent to which the different blades of the pin-wheel share business, clinical, and economic risk with other blades. The index categorizes four main components of this part of the index. In case you forgot, just color in the pie slices.

Q#1   Payor (carrier) bears full risk: do not record

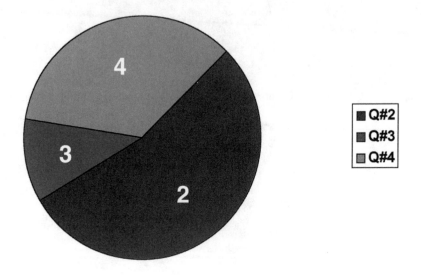

Q#2   Payor shares risk with physician

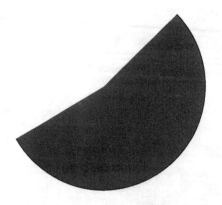

Q#3   Payor shares risk with hospital

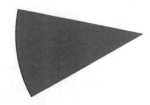

Q#4   Shared risk among payor, hospital, and physicians

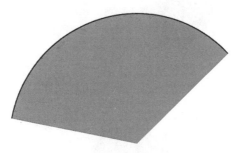

In 1993, The Institute of the Future estimated very little risk sharing among providers, as follows:

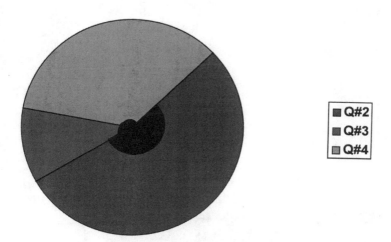

Again, for those in the research planning professions, the baseline index metrics are presented in Appendix B. We still have a way to go, but at the very least we have established a beachhead of research upon which we can build over the next few years.

The Managed-Care Index At-A-Glance

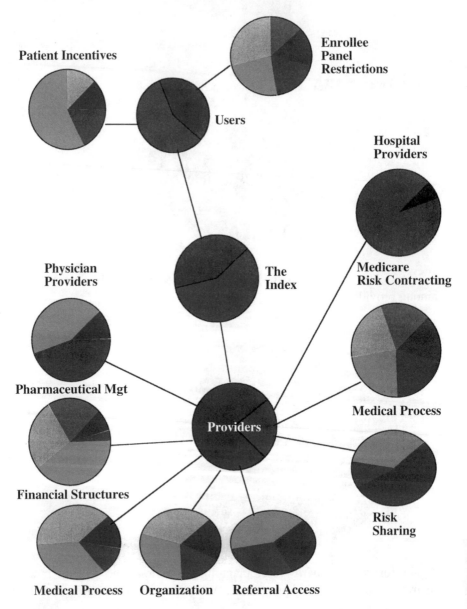

THE JOURNEY FROM LITE TO HEAVY

This introduction to the managed-care index merely a brief introduction. As we indexers actually go about tracking managed-care presence over time, we should continuously upgrade our methods for assessing where a market stands and where it is likely headed. A static methodology that inscribes its scores in stone can be of no use whatsoever in today's rapidly changing environment. We need moving pictures, not snapshots.

Conscientious managed-care indexers must also continuously expand the number of indicators they regularly study. Back in the early 1980s, when the industry first recognized that managed care was a phenomenon worth tracking, one just looked at the number of people enrolled in federally qualified HMOs or state-licensed prepaid health plans. These days, our industry's major health plans, hospital systems, and medical groups follow a broad array of data elements and prevailing trends. Already the indicators, scales, survey questions, and baseline estimates listed previously betray the ever-expanding aspirations of this indexing tool. With each passing month, it seems, planners understand better the marketplace forces that will affect their businesses. One's understanding of these shaping forces must ever blossom as a marketplace evolves.

Especially important will be the ability to detect the "friction point" in market development, when a region begins its transition out of the lite environment and enters a glidepath into the world of fully managed care. Health plans, hospital systems, and medical groups each must grow to understand and anticipate its own milestones along the road from managed-care lite to managed-care heavy. My clients and colleagues in positions of authority at major HMOs, health plans, hospitals, integrated delivery systems, large medical groups, and specialty physician practices have shared some of the indicators they will be watching over the years ahead.

HMOs and Health Plans

Beyond the overall HMO penetration or share of the market's commercial and Medicare populations, already incorporated in comprehensive managed-care indexing, many of today's more astute health maintenance organizations and major health plans also track: the unionization of the area workforce, because unions do tend to favor managed care; the percentage of business channeled through insurance brokers; the premium structures and benefits of the most representative employer benefits plans;

and the proclivities of leaders on the provider side, including any big medical groups that enjoy name recognition and a high-quality image as well as growing hospital systems that may soon become friends or foes.

The index can handily signal the friction point where the payor community emerges into a managed-care heavy market. Often we see a frenzy of physician contracting just before the friction point, which upon closer inspection may be nothing more than a heated competition among financing agencies who are delivering volume and cutting deals with the same providers. In more mature markets, observant HMOs and health plans have learned that providers become increasingly divided, clustered, and linked with financing or health plan mechanisms. Then, as the market fragments, market shares consolidate. Three to five managed-care players soon control the member population and, in order to maintain the affordability and effectiveness of care, grow quite competitive. Over the long term, these health plans want to get their arms around the delivery system side of the business, through contracts, through partnerships, or by any variety of aggressive measures.

For HMOs and health plans several managed-care milestones deserve special attention. A managed-care lite market is characterized by delivery systems walled off from one another. Things start getting heavy when market shares consolidate, health plans compete head to head and begin to acquire or partner with provider systems, and delivery models grow more and more sophisticated, that is, integrated by contract.

Hospitals and Health Networks

Time was, a bricks-and-mortar healthcare organization was glad just to win some guaranteed patient volume from the market's fledgling managed-care plans. Finally, hospitals and health networks are beginning to understand the risks they bear and have started asking the right questions. What major health plans am I dealing with, and how many members are in each? What are the relationships between the plans and their subscribers? Are the plans strictly conduits for money, or are they genuinely striving to adjust service delivery to meet the needs of the populations they serve?

The money-conduit plans quickly resort to police tactics, such as retroactive denials, limitations of service, and strict adherence to numbers and guidelines that leave precious little room for human judgment. All these techniques have become primary targets of the managed-care backlash. Real care-managing plans define their populations and work to serve the healthcare needs of those members, attaining cost-effectiveness without merely wielding economic bludgeons against providers and subscribers.

Providers can most reliably monitor their own level of capitation to signal the friction point between managed-care lite and managed-care heavy. When they are aggressively acquiring practice management companies on the physician side, providers look for medical groups that are committed to managed care and already have more than half of their business capitated. As one of my trusted colleagues puts it, capitation is the provider's surest bellwether for managed care, because it sets all the incentives right and the utilization review becomes your friend and not your enemy. In short, the managed-care market really falls into place when providers are put at risk for their own behaviors.

Provider executives of my long acquaintance have noted certain shortcomings of the managed-care index. What might happen, some have asked me, if the index were constructed to profile the risk of caring for different age groups under certain disease categories and stages? What many also miss is the whole notion of integrated care which is widely considered the highest form of managed care. I agree. The real test of any managed-care organization is the capacity to ask, What are we actually doing to improve care and improve the health of our population? The index's current indicators for organizational structure of physician practice settings, hospital integration of medicine, and risk sharing do capture some but not all of the indicators of integrated delivery across the marketplace. Some providers have also observed that the index lacks a subacute component to gauge the shift out of traditional facilities and sickness models. And it should further consider, others argue, how plans and providers work together to weigh the tradeoffs and decide upon a care location.

Of course I welcome these criticisms of the managed-care index. After all, this tool is necessarily a work in progress, as is the healthcare marketplace it endeavors to portray. I fully intend to enhance the model as my clients and readers demonstrate the inclination and the wherewithal to gather and interpret additional pieces of vital planning information. I invite the readers to send their comments and suggestions to me at my e-mail address DennisPatterson1@Compuserve.com.

Large Medical Groups

Physician organizations have become bona fide managed-care entities and forces to be reckoned with. Most of all, big medical groups want to know precisely how much risk is actually pushed down to the provider level, and how much is kept at the plan level. In California providers might bear global risk, whereas on the Eastern Seaboard very little risk gets passed down to the provider level. In many markets the health plans have retained all the risk themselves, remaining content to just pay discounted fees for services to the physicians and the hospitals.

A medical group at the friction point of managed-care heavy stands ready and willing to accept full global risk, not only on the professional side but on the institutional and pharmacy side as well. In order to achieve the best management of care, planners know the group needs to wield overall control. A sophisticated group might first track how much of its business is capitated for each segment, that is, professional, institutional, and pharmaceutical and then try to push toward global risk out of those parameters.

One physician group executive distinguishes lite from heavy as follows:

- A managed-care lite market has embraced no global risk concepts, in which hospitals earn per diems and HMOs have retained all the hospital risk. They enforce some primary care capitation, but probably a very small percentage of the full professional cap; the market is under perhaps 20% full professional cap. Medical process management is in the infant stage, still using a strong gatekeeper model to control the specialist side and driving the hospital days down to the 220 range.

- A managed-care heavy market has about 60% global risk and has driven medical management up to the next level. Hospital days are down to 170 or lower. The referral process is practically automatic; nobody thinks twice about making the right physician referral. And nobody has to wait a week to get one; by the time you leave the primary care office you have got a referral and you are scheduled to see a specialist.

Speaking of specialists, they have a unique perspective on the journey from managed-care lite to heavy. Most specialists with national experience do not really consider it a managed-care market unless large provider groups have been capitated or accepted some form of prepaid moneys. Perhaps in the near future we will see spot capitation markets that still use fee-for-service for certain segments of their product but use capitation for specialists and perhaps hospitals.

According to specialty practice groups, a managed-care lite market has high bed days, one or two HMOs or so-called HMO products, an over-abundance of specialists, and not very well integrated specialties. There is a fair amount of managed-care competition, that is, capitated insurance products penetrating 20% of the market or more. Managed competition equals health, the specialist feels, and many would like to see four to nine HMOs in a given metropolitan service area.

As the managed-care heavy market approaches, the specialist observes, first comes a greater capitation of specialists and then a greater capitation of hospitals. When about 25% of the healthcare insurance products in a given service area are prepaid and capitated, hospitals will start sharing the risk as fast as they can sign the contracts. This is a golden opportunity for hospitals to get their revenue streams flowing, if they can work smart and learn to play the game. In California, our hospitals are absolutely begging to be capitated. Who would have imagined that just three years ago! They want to be capitated so they can win volume, because they understand that volume is the game now. The hospital's strategy should be, first, to capture as much capitation as it can to secure the volume of specialist panels and, second, to adjust its own costs so it can make some money off that newfound capitated business.

SUMMARY

In concept, in design, and in practical use, the managed-care index presents a daunting challenge for a new breed of healthcare strategist. Somehow our capacity for change must keep pace with the market. Somehow our stores of meaningful, fresh data must remain as rich as the exciting new opportunity to truly manage the health of vast populations. The index is but our latest and brightest hope for answering these challenges. This chapter and the next constitute a "kit" for strategists to craft a tool that can support tough decisions by most accurately measuring the market presence and advancement of managed care.

Skilled managed-care indexers may well enjoy a clear view of their marketplaces at-a-glance, but good peripheral vision will prove just as important in piloting the managed-care transformation. Look about and consider the viewpoints of others in the marketplace and across your pinwheel. For vigilant payors, providers, and physicians alike, the journey from managed-care lite to managed-care heavy promises adventure at every turn. A reliable compass like the managed-care index might come in handy.

6
CHAPTER

Gathering Information and Calibrating the Index

Unlike other, conventional interpretations of healthcare's ongoing market evolution, the managed-care index is designed to quantify the true managed-care presence in a marketplace. Immediate predecessors of the managed-care indexing methodology merely counted HMO enrollees, divided by the total population, multiplied by one hundred, and called that percentage "market penetration." But you cannot simply ask members for a show of hands and reasonably conclude that they will tell you how much healthcare your market now manages. The true management of care and health, we have learned in preceding chapters, only just begins when a member enrolls in a health plan.

Any accurate and meaningful measure of managed-care presence must chiefly account for the observable managed-care *actions* and likely *consequences* among both providers and users in a marketplace. So managed-care indexing takes a closer look at who the real managed-care players are and what they are really doing to influence one another's behavior. Each sector of the marketplace must be viewed as both actor and reactor; that is, a managed-care index of proper scope describes influential activities and natural reactions throughout the marketplace by gathering vital data across the full span of the managed-care pinwheel. Only then can planners calculate an index score that will reliably inform the benchmarking strategies promised in the subtitle of this book.

The fully calibrated managed-care index, as introduced in Chapter 5, incorporates data that quantify the following ten different clinical and business practices that influence every other provider and user in the marketplace, namely:

- Patient managed-care incentives;
- Enrollee provider panel restrictions;
- Process management of pharmaceuticals;
- Physician financial structures;
- Medical process management of physicians;
- Organizational structure of physician practice setting;
- Physician referral access;
- Medicare risk contracting percentage;
- Hospital medical process management; and
- Risk sharing among hospitals, physicians, and payors.

Add to this list the general level of acceptance among patients and physicians, quite easily and adequately gleaned via unscientific surveys, and you have a pretty complete picture of what makes a managed-care market tick.

Knowing where to find such data and keeping a fresh supply always on hand must become a core planning discipline of the managed-care organization. The three Cs rule this new discipline of managed-care indexing, and they are comparative, comprehensive, and composited. The robust indexing process taps the most reliable comparative databases, gathers all the essential data elements, subjects those raw data to rigorous analysis, and composites the results in one easy-to-read report with easy-to-understand scores.

This chapter considers the various sources and techniques used to compile raw market information. It further explains how to calculate an overall score of managed-care presence using the index's sophisticated but practical system of scales and weights, through which essential survey results, comparative data, key statistics, and empirical information are rendered strategically meaningful.

CONSIDER THE SOURCE

A sound managed-care indexing methodology rests on a firm foundation of both quantitative and qualitative benchmarks, based on reliable information about the users and providers in your healthcare marketplace. Unfortunately, gathering even the most rudimentary benchmark data can be a formidable challenge in the present environment. No single source of comprehensive managed-care data is available as of this writing. Soon enough, within this book's shelf life, several clearinghouses will emerge to offer the diligent indexer a wide selection of truly comprehensive data packages.

Yet there is no good reason for the resourceful healthcare organization to wait until the perfect one-stop store of knowledge arrives. Already several rich sources of national, regional, and local market information can provide much of the raw data required to calculate your managed-care index.

As explained in Chapter 5, the managed-care index compiles and weighs data from managed-care users (enrollees and patients) and providers (physicians, hospitals, and pharmacies) to arrive at an overall index score. In this chapter we suggest potential data sources for these component parts of the managed-care index.

Please note that some of the data provided by the organizations noted here may be proprietary and, in many cases, costly. Whenever vital information is too hard to come by or too expensive to acquire, I recommend that my clients roll up their sleeves and, with proper guidance and advice, design instruments to collect their own data and conduct their own surveys. In addition, many of the data sources noted provide Internet web sites for public use and any World Wide Web search engine should help make the connection for you.

Again, the flexibility to make or buy all the raw information you need is fast becoming a core discipline of good strategic planning. The following sources should become accomplished pieces in the basic repertoire of data gathering and analysis.

COMPILING INFORMATION ABOUT USERS

Learning precisely how consumers (enrollees and patients) are reacting to the managed-care phenomenon and, moreover, exerting their own influence in your marketplace is job number one. Besides enrollees and patients, the user group should be understood to include the employers and benefits managers who, in the final analysis, shape the employee's choice of healthcare coverage.

Managed-care indexing captures user behavior in two indicators: patient managed-care incentives and enrollee provider panel restrictions.

Developing a firm grasp of *patient managed-care incentives* will require information on the number of uninsured in your marketplace, the average level of deductibles and co-payments, and common types of restrictions on and financial incentives for using specific provider panels. Understanding the influential role of *enrollee provider panel restrictions* will require an analysis of information about the use of primary-care physician gatekeepers, the percentage of utilization outside of provider networks, and various additional information about the provider panels themselves. Several data sources, foremost among them the organizations listed as follows, can provide such data for all users, both enrollees and patients.

- Summary data—The Employee Benefit Research Institute (EBRI) is a nonprofit, nonpartisan policy research organization based in Washington, DC. The Institute produces and distributes a wide range of publications concerning health, welfare, and retirement policies including invaluable summary data on the insured and uninsured populations in the nation as well as more general information about the way health protection in our country has changed.

- Premiums, deductibles, and co-payments—The Health Care Financing Administration (HCFA), headquartered in Baltimore, MD, oversees national Medicare policy relating, administers the program, and oversees states' administration of Medicaid. Premium, deductible, and co-payment data is typically available through the state rate filings with the Department of Insurance or similar regulatory department.

- HMO enrollment—InterStudy Publications, located in Minneapolis/St. Paul, MN, conducts research and publishes reports on the HMO industry, managed-care topics, and quality and information management in healthcare. InterStudy maintains perhaps the best longitudinal database on HMO enrollment trends.

- Plan selection—The American Association of Health Plans (AAHP) (formerly Group Health Association of America, American Managed Care and Review Association) in Washington, DC, conducts research and reports digested information about the managed-care industry. In 1996 the AAHP developed and administered an annual survey to over 2400 health plans that offer HMO and/or PPO products. The results of this survey, which asked the respondents to describe their products, contracted providers, level of financial risk, enrollment, plan characteristics, benefits, premiums, co-payments, deductibles, and other plan information, will be available in years following through the AAHP's Data and Resource Center.

COMPILING INFORMATION ABOUT PROVIDERS

In delivering virtually all healthcare services, technologies, and supplies, the healthcare providers (physicians, hospitals, and pharmacies) wield perhaps the most control over the managed-care landscape. These provider entities should be understood to include the large group medical practices, health systems, and pharmaceutical benefits management firms that have been so influential as of late.

Physicians

In managed-care indexing, the five indicators, process management of pharmaceuticals, physician financial structures, medical process management, organizational structure of physician practice setting, and physician referral access, capture the behavior of physicians in the managed-care marketplace. These indicators focus on characteristics of physician practice structures and financial incentives as well as certain aspects of process management, such as the management of pharmaceuticals and the medical management of patients.

The information provided by today's available sources of physician practice data may not be as comprehensive as the data available for the other index components. A survey of local area physician groups may sometimes be an easier and more reliable alternative to the following sources listed.

- Practice information—The American Medical Association (AMA), headquartered in Chicago, IL, continues to develop its comprehensive database of physician and medical student information (AMA Masterfile). The two AMA-administered surveys, Physician Census and Socioeconomic Monitoring System, include information particularly relevant to the managed-care index. The AMA's Data Survey and Planning Department and/or the Center for Health Policy Research can assist in the gathering of physician demographics, socioeconomic characteristics, and other practice information.

- Medical group management—The United Medical Group Association (UMGA) in Seal Beach, CA, provides a broad range of data on group practice leadership and professional development, education, credentialing, information processing, communication, advocacy, networking, and research activities. The majority of the Association's research is centered on medical group management issues. The UMGA administers annual member surveys on national standards for medical practice. State-by-state data from the survey is available, including type of group, ownership, number of physicians, percentage of managed care, and other medical group characteristics.

- Reimbursement—InterStudy Publications gathers information on provider reimbursement as part of its annual survey of HMOs. An annual industry report looks at various methods of reimbursement (including capitation, fee-for-service, relative value scale, DRG, per diem, and salary) for primary-care physicians, specialty-care physicians, and hospitals. Detailed information is available through InterStudy analysts.

Hospitals

In managed-care indexing, the three indicators, Medicare risk contracting, hospital process management, and risk sharing capture the behaviors of hospitals in a managed-care marketplace. Data requirements include information on the market penetration of Medicare risk products, the level of process management in area hospitals, and risk sharing arrangements between health plans, physicians, and hospitals.

Again, it may sometimes be easier and more reliable to survey local providers to attain this information, aside from Medicare penetration data, which are easily available through HCFA. Recommended sources for the hospital components of the index are as follows:

- Medicare risk—The Health Care Financing Administration, as previously noted, is responsible for gathering information regarding Medicare beneficiaries, including those enrolled in risk products. HCFA publishes a monthly "Medicare Managed-Care Contract Report" that provides comprehensive information on Medicare eligibles, beneficiaries, and risk enrollees, by state.

More detailed information is available through HCFA's central office. This information and the annual AAPCC (average adjusted per capita cost) figures are also accessible electronically via the HCFA web site, www.hcfa.gov.

- Process management and risk sharing—The American Hospital Association (AHA) conducts an Annual Survey of Hospitals that seeks a variety of information, not all of which is published in the AHA guidebooks. Data is generally provided by the Health Care Information Resources Group.

- Overall performance—Officed in Baltimore, MD, the healthcare information firm HCIA Inc. develops clinical and financial decision-making support systems and markets them to hospitals, integrated delivery systems, managed-care organizations, and pharmaceutical manufacturers. HCIA profiles available information on the financial, operational, and clinical performance of nearly all American hospitals, using more than 50 performance measures.

- Reimbursement—InterStudy Publications, as previously noted, gathers information on provider reimbursement as part of its annual survey of HMOs.

- Impanelment—The American Association of Health Plans, as previously noted, has begun administering an annual survey of its member organizations to collect information on their products, contracted providers, levels of financial risk, enrollment, plan characteristics, benefits, premiums, co-payments and deductibles, and other plan information. The survey results will be available through AAHP's Data and Resource Center.

CALCULATING INDEX WEIGHTS, SCALES, AND SCORES

Perhaps the best way to demonstrate how the components of the managed-care index are properly weighed and scaled is to explain once again how Dr. Ian Morrison and I originally conceived the index. We, our colleagues, and selected advisors first established key indicators of managed-care presence, agreed to graduated scales for each indicator, gathered all the context data we could gather, and combined those numbers with the best estimates from the Institute for the Future think tank. Then we assembled an expert panel to reality-test our indicators and weights and, having devised an overall index scoring procedure supported by weighed calculation worksheets for each indicator, fed the whole thing into our untested model.

The results showed a national managed-care presence just over 20% (20.44 to be exact), which fit nicely with our experience and expectations back in 1993. This initial scoring exercise helped calibrate the first index according to the best available national data.

Figure 6–1, the Managed-Care Index "Fishbone," affords a complete overview of all the indicators that feed into the calculation of index scores. Tables 6–1 through 6–9 show how to calculate weights and index contributions for each of the indicators, using our own 1993 numbers as a proxy.

FIGURE 6–1

The Managed-Care Index "Fishbone"

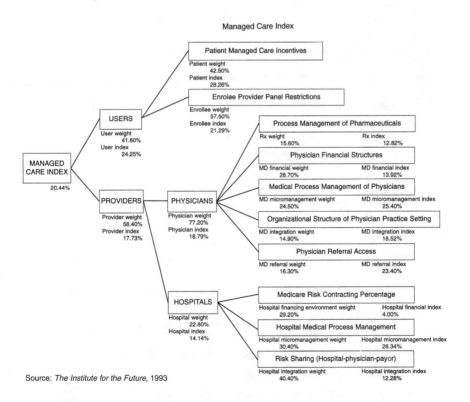

Source: *The Institute for the Future,* 1993

TABLE 6-1

Index Calculation Worksheet:
Patient Managed-Care Incentives

	Share of Total	Contribution	Weight	Index
No health insurance	14%	0%	0	28.26%
Insured with deductible under $100	7%	3%	0.00217	
Insured with deductible/copayment $100-$200	7%	10%	0.007	
Insured with deductible/copayment above $200	8%	14%	0.01136	
Insured, but subject to 1 or more of:			0	
Share with at least two on the above list	22%	21%	0.04576	
Share with at least four on the above list	14%	30%	0.04158	
Share with at least six on the above list	5%	40%	0.01985	
Financial incentive to use restricted panel (ranging from 1%-10%)	5%	45%	0.0223	
Financial incentive to use restricted panel (ranging from 11-29%)	5%	56%	0.0282	
Financial incentive to use restricted panel (30-99%)	4%	68%	0.02728	
Restricted panel for primary care	4%	77%	0.03084	
Restricted panel for all medical care	4%	91%	0.0362	
Restricted panel for all healthcare (including other professionals such as mental health, drug abuse, and optometrist; and other needs such as diagnostic tests and pharmaceuticals).	1%	100%	0.01001	
TOTAL	100%			

Source: *The Institute for the Future,* 1993

Ten carefully scaled and weighed marketplace indicators constitute the overall index score:

- Patient managed-care incentives (Table 6–1);
- Enrollee provider panel restrictions (Table 6–2);
- Process management of pharmaceuticals (Table 6–3);
- Physician financial structures (Table 6–4);

TABLE 6-2

Index Calculation Worksheet:
Enrollee Provider Panel Restrictions

	Population	Contribution	Weighted Value	Index
No restrictions	55%	0%	0	25.44%
Network, 10% or less to go outside	10%	17%	0.0174	
Network, 11% or more to go outside	16%	35%	0.0552	
Network with gatekeeper, up to 29% copayment	1%	58%	0.00584	
Network with gatekeeper, 30% or more copayment	3%	87%	0.02598	
Closed panel w/o POS	15%	100%	0.15	
TOTAL	100%			

Source: *The Institute for the Future*, 1993

- Medical process management of physicians (Table 6–5);
- Organizational structure of physician practice setting (Table 6–6);
- Physician referral access (Table 6–7);
- Medicare risk contracting (calculated as a pure percentage of Medicare lives under contract);
- Hospital medical process management (Table 6–8); and
- Risk sharing among hospitals, physicians, and payors (Table 6–9).

We chose these indicators to capture, as comprehensively as possible, the real dynamics of the managed-care marketplace. The composite score thus portrays how all the various players are acting to influence other providers and users in a given marketplace.

Here is a fine beginning, anyway. You can use the fishbone diagram (Fig. 6–1) and calculation worksheets (Tables 6–1 through 6–9) as a template to custom design a managed-care index for your own marketplace. Rather than prescribing a closed menu of sources to tap, I suggest that planners rely on the information they understand the best and trust the most. Rather than outlining a strict indexing methodology to follow, I suggest you make it specific, make it relevant, and make it personal. A tailored approach stands the fairest chance of lasting success.

TABLE 6-3

Index Calculation Worksheet:
Process Management of Pharmaceuticals

	Physicians	Contribution	Weighted Value	Index
No restrictions on prescribing	58%	0%	0	12.82%
Lite MC, no review	8%	7%	0.00528	
Heavy MC, no review	13%	12%	0.01573	
Lite MC, pharma review	7%	36%	0.02541	
Heavy MC, pharma review	13%	57%	0.07423	
Lite MC, MD review	1%	76%	0.00759	
Heavy MC, MD review	0%	100%	0	
TOTAL	100%			

Source: *The Institute for the Future,* 1993

TABLE 6-4

Index Calculation Worksheet:
Physician Financial Structures

	Patients	Contribution	Weighted Value	Index
Unmanaged FFS	7%	0%	0	15.79%
Discounted FFS	68%	8%	0.05168	
FFS w/risk pool	13%	12%	0.01534	
Cap (primary care only)	4%	52%	0.02092	
Cap (specialty)	5%	.78.7	0.04	
Global capitation	3%	100%	0.03	
TOTAL	100%			

Source: *The Institute for the Future,* 1993

TABLE 6 – 5

Index Calculation Worksheet:
Medical Process Management of Physicians

	Physicians	Contribution	Weighted Value	Index
No process management	24%	0%	0	25.40%
Light utiliz. review	38%	15%	0.05814	
Light process management	20%	27%	0.0548	
Heavy process management	10%	61%	0.0611	
"Cultural controls" (incl. heavy process management)	8%	100%	0.08	
TOTAL	100%			

Source: *The Institute for the Future*, 1993

TABLE 6 – 6

Index Calculation Worksheet:
Organizational Structure of Physician Practice Settings

	Physicians	Contribution	Weighted Value	Index
Independent practice	65%	0%	0	18.52%
Single-specialty group practice	15%	20%	0.03	
Small multi-specialty group	5%	37%	0.0183	
Medium multi-specialty group	4%	67%	0.02692	
Large multi-specialty group	11%	100%	0.11	
TOTAL	100%			

Source: *The Institute for the Future*, 1993

TABLE 6-7

Index Calculation Worksheet:
Physician Referral Access

	Patients	Contribution	Weighted Value	Index
No restrictions	42.00%	0.00%	0.00	23.42%
PPO (general restrictions)	48.00%	30.50%	0.15	
Closed panel restrictions (some specialties)	3.00%	59.20%	0.02	
Closed panel restrictions (all specialties)	7.00%	100.00%	0.07	
TOTAL	100.00%			

Source: *The Institute for the Future,* 1993

TABLE 6-8

Index Calculation Worksheet:
Hospital Medical Process Management

	Patients	Contribution	Weighted Value	Index
No restrictions	25%	0%	0	26.34%
Pre-admission certification (only)	29%	17%	0.04814	
Discharge planning	28%	37%	0.10444	
Concurrent utilization review (case management)	17%	60%	0.10268	
Detailed practice guidelines or critical pathways	1%	82%	0.00818	
Clinical CQI/TQM	0%	100%	0	
TOTAL	100%			

Source: *The Institute for the Future,* 1993

TABLE 6-9

Index Calculation Worksheet:
Risk Sharing, Hospital-Physician-Payor

	Patients	Contribution	Weighted Value	Index
Payor (carrier) has risk	81%	0%	0	12.28%
Payor shares risk	10%	54%	0.0538	
Payor shares risk with hospital	6%	65%	0.039	
Shared risk between payor, hospital, and physician	3%	100%	0.03	
TOTAL	100%			

Source: The Institute for the Future, 1993

   Please also refer back to the indexing sections of Chapter 5 and to Appendix B for further details on the scale of activities we considered, possible survey questions, and original Institute for the Future estimates that helped us calibrate the model and design and refine this managed-care index. Combined with up-to-date information from the numerous sources listed in this chapter, these tools give managed-care indexers everything they need to calibrate the model and calculate a meaningful and useful measure of managed-care presence. Again, I invite your ideas and suggestions to my e-mail address at DennisPatterson1@Compuserve.com.

   Together, Chapters 5 and 6 (plus the two related Appendixes) also offer a sneak preview of a forthcoming indexing tool featuring strategic benchmarks collected from distinguished national, regional, and local sources. More to the point, the figures and worksheets assembled in this section should help you understand the indexing basics and inspire you to imagine what the complete managed-care index might look like. To be of any practical use, this entire managed-care indexing process must be carefully designed and put to good work for your very own organization and local market. The time is ripe for every healthcare organization to learn how to select reliable sources, gather the essential data, properly analyze the bits and numbers, and translate it all into digestible information. Such is the plain language in which today's healthcare planner must demonstrate fluency.

7
CHAPTER

Putting the Index to Good Work

Now that you are familiar with the various pieces of information you will have to gather for managed-care indexing, and now that you understand how those pieces, all together, can help you gauge the presence of managed-care in your marketplace, the time has come to assemble the puzzle and admire the big picture.

Once the appropriate data have been compiled and your managed-care index is fully calibrated, strategists must next learn how to put the index to work as a reliable benchmarking tool and a solid foundation for future planning. A beginner's guide to interpreting and applying the information produced through managed-care indexing, this chapter dispenses a bit of practical advice regarding how all the components of a healthcare market, that is providers, physician groups, and payors together can outfit themselves strategically for the stepwise journey from managed-care lite to managed-care heavy.

The journey progresses in varying speeds, because managed-care market penetration has a curiously cumulative effect. Among my own client organizations I have noticed that those in lite markets, posting an index score lower than 20% or so, kind of play-act their way through managed-care. Of course they read all the journals, too, and have learned to emulate convincingly the habits and speech patterns of real managed-care practitioners. Once the market breaks through that 30% wall, though, the pantomime ends. The market takes off like a rocket and the full throttle of managed care carries the field up to an index score of 60% in no time.

Somewhere along the line, you see, a marketplace begins to drive its own transformation, whether on the strength of employee acceptance, cost differential, or price elasticity. Even the most reform-averse factions start to adapt to managed care, then begrudgingly accept it and get with the program. Fear soon dissipates. The best-laid plans of provider, physician, and payor organizations find their mark.

PROVIDER STRATEGIES

For healthcare providers, who own the community's bricks-and-mortar assets and operate the programs those facilities house, the first order of business is to use the index to develop a deeper understanding of your organization's position in its marketplace. Does your executive team actually possess the ability to set a strategy that will allow the organization to keep pace with its payors, as they migrate from managed-care lite to managed-care heavy?

Too often we see payors invading unsophisticated markets wielding all-too-sophisticated managed-care techniques, much to the detriment of the payors, their memberships, and providers alike. On the other hand, payors are not always the aggressors. Providers should be careful not to get too far ahead of the payors, either.

I find that providers who are ready to accept capitation today, or eager to consider partnership arrangements in which they would bear considerable risk, have jumped well ahead of payors in many markets. To keep in step with the market, all along the winding pathway from managed-care lite to managed-care heavy, providers may have to adopt then abruptly jettison any number of different strategies. Most important, a provider organization must set the tone among its own managers and rank-and-file workers, creating an expectation that "together we are going to migrate as the market migrates from managed-care lite to managed-care heavy."

Strategic Multiplicity and Medical Staff Relations

For probably the first time in the history of healthcare, today's provider has no choice but to juggle multiple strategies and substrategies. A hospital or health system might wisely craft distinct strategies for its fee-for-service, center-of-excellence, charity, indemnity, government, and managed-care lines of business, any of which may involve some but not all of its specialists. Adhering to the pinwheel concept, a hospital would do well to concentrate on handling its own continuum of care as the market becomes more saturated with managed-care lines.

Before leaping into a diversified portfolio of targeted strategies, planners must consider the effect on medical staff relationships. The traditional institution manager strives to include everyone in every strategy. But in a capitated environment, winning broad physician participation too early is perhaps the surest way to kill a fledgling planning effort, because so many physicians bristle at the very thought of bearing or sharing risk. Physicians who have enjoyed years and years of lucrative medical practices in the meat and potato days of fee-for-service reimbursement can prove to be especially reluctant, or even combative, partners in the salad days of managed care.

As the organization migrates from managed-care lite to managed-care heavy, the crux of the medical staff matter is to fully understand the number of specialists you will need in order to service the populations for which you sign risk contracts. Over time, as those contractual relationships and covered lives are channeled to a few individual practitioners, a provider and its medical staff learn how to operate in a managed-care environment.

So even an institution in a managed-care lite market, serving very few covered lives, would be smart to pilot its initial managed-care efforts among a small cadre of specialists. As such efforts bloom and grow into predominant marketplace strategies, doctors can teach doctors how they have learned to operate with providers in a managed-care environment.

Volume, Volume, Volume

Rookie managed-care providers most commonly stumble over volume. If you cannot amass enough managed-care volume to gain the attention of specialists, you can hardly expect them to change their behaviors or practice patterns, nor will the institution have the proper incentive to change. Insufficient volume will give your new managed-care operation the wonderful ability to lose money at an ever-accelerating rate.

Another surefire way the new managed-care provider can throw away money is by diffusing its initial managed-care focus beyond a small cadre of dedicated physicians. As the market and the institution proceed from lite to heavy, a core group of specialists can devote their undivided attention to cultivating the managed-care strategy and learning how physicians and hospitals can manage clinical and business risk and win. A more ambitious rollout plan, involving a broader cross-section of physicians, some of whom might only dabble in managed care, will more likely just propagate a weak cost structure that had been losing a little bit on each managed-care case. Then, as managed care penetration becomes greater, all those little losses quickly add up until they absolutely devastate your bottom line.

Often we see provider institutions sign away their souls at the going risk-capitation rate, because they reckon that sooner or later payors will drive providers' volume anyway, and if providers do not act now they will later be coerced into accepting risk at bargain-basement prices. Why not face the music and join the dance on one's own terms? But it is foolhardy to jump right into a managed-care heavy market strategy without ever having gone through the baby steps of learning how to deal with changing care delivery in a managed-care lite market.

Virtuality and the Exploding Care Continuum

As the bricks-and-mortar sector of the healthcare community evolves from a managed-care lite into a managed-care heavy frame of mind, the walls come tumbling down. Hospitals and health systems move beyond merely controlling processes within the four walls of the traditional healthcare institution and start looking around the pinwheel to grasp the full continuum of care. Home health, long-term care, rehabilitative care, and even social services contracts become ever more important planks in the strategic platform of the emerging managed-care provider.

But no central institution need own every program and building in the system to offer a comprehensive array of services; the full continuum of care may be assembled and maintained just as effectively through contractual arrangements. The superior flexibility of such virtual arrangements becomes more and more critical as you move from a discounted fee-for-service to per diem, to per case, and eventually to capitation rates.

Executive leaders at the system level are then challenged to cultivate a new thought process among managers and physicians at every organizational level and site of care. The sensitive question everyone should be asking is, How best can we move this patient along, as soon as clinically appropriate, from intensive care to acute care, to rehabilitation, to long-term care, to home, so that the patient gets just the right care and the case rate turns a profit for the lead institution and for all the other players in the continuum of care? Why treat a patient in an acute care setting, just out of habit or for the sake of tradition, when that patient's health can be restored more quickly or even initially in a subacute facility, in some kind of ambulatory care setting, in a physician's office, or right at home?

For providers, a management philosophy that constantly and intelligently questions the appropriateness of the care setting is the hallmark of sound managed-care practice. Failing to adopt such a philosophy in time will render a hospital or health system strategically immobile and, as payors off-load their responsibility for medical loss ratios via capitated rates, providers will drown in risk. Do not concentrate on the bed, concentrate on the member.

PHYSICIAN GROUP STRATEGIES

Whether practicing in primary care networks or in multispecialty care networks, doctors face several complicating factors as they follow the market from managed-care lite to managed-care heavy. Again one has to recognize that, whenever a managed-care organization enters a new marketplace, its chief desire is to include as many outstanding physicians and reputable institutions as possible in the network listing. The employer is customer number one, and the plan wants to make a good first impression that it can service anyone in the market.

But as the market matures, the only way a payor can continue to offer employers a decreasing premium is to gain tighter control over its network. Of course it works to the payor's distinct advantage if it can manage to deliver superior and convenient service through a smaller network, while maintaining enough volume to attract the attention of physicians.

Volume, Volume, Volume

My earlier warning for a bricks-and-mortar philosophy also holds true for physicians where insufficient volume will give your physician group's new managed-care operation the wonderful ability to lose money at an ever-accelerating rate. During the initial penetration of managed care, we often witness physician groups scrambling to form Independent Practice Associations (IPAs). But in their rush to service all the payor groups that are entering the market and reserve a seat in those broad networks, physicians seldom pause to notice that the new plans drive very little, if any, additional volume through to the individual physicians they sign up.

Groups caught up in the market whirlwind, with one eye fixed on the perfect future and the other on their wallets, might even stop concentrating on the essential medical responsibilities at hand. Clinical decision making and individual patient treatment sometimes wane in the early stages of managed care. It is a completely understandable but certainly not acceptable state of affairs when the contemporary managed-care physician, justifiably worried about the survival of his or her own enterprise, is apt to be distracted by extraclinical matters, like whether the payors' incentives regarding referral patterns, utilization reviews, prior authorization, and such are just too much of a hassle.

As the Dust Settles

Early on, physicians can be either too eager to join up or too cautious to change. They openly dare health plan champions to prove that managed care is something more than a nuisance and something less than a threat to the health of their valued patients and to the future of their livelihoods.

In due course, as the market matures from managed-care lite to managed-care heavy, physician groups can gain an acceptable level of comfort and control. Today the more successful medical groups, in the most mature markets, are taking a boldly confident strategic tack. Some are actually controlling their networks, either through formal contracts or through incentive relationships, in such a way that they can accept full capitation from payors. In the California market, at least two major medical groups have gone so far as to accept a limited HMO license, so that they can now accept a fully capitated rate from *any* payor. Such a strategy clearly aims to control the memberships of all payors so the group can negotiate the best possible rate with all the institutions that it will funnel its covered populations.

More important, perhaps, these physicians are pioneers in learning precisely how to deliver the best member service at the most appropriate cost, which is an absolutely essential development for a healthcare system in which primary care and specialty physicians control about 80% of total costs. But even in mature markets, let us remember, strict managed care still constitutes only a few chapters in the average physician's book of business. Patient bases these days still have traditional indemnity policies and, increasingly, on alternative managed-care products, like point-of-service options, which retain the look and feel of indemnity policies.

Payors are starting to become aware of how completely these larger medical groups wield control over their members, and some payors have started to contemplate the day when physician groups can contract directly with employers.

Eyes on the Pinwheel: Good Doctors Make Bad Insurers

Even the very boldest physician initiatives need not be out of step with the pinwheel concept, under which hospitals, payors, and physicians stick to running their own businesses and stop dabbling in other parts of the industry. I believe that our more sophisticated medical groups, even those who have begun to take on capitation, do fully understand that some underwriting and marketing functions, especially concerning membership service and satisfaction, are best handled by an insurance function.

Physician groups make poor insurers. And hospital executives who believe that, merely by joint venturing with their physicians, they can go directly to employers, will find it tough to put such beliefs into action. Despite having demonstrated an admirable capability to work in conjunction with its physicians, no one superprovider can manage the whole underwriting function, run a top-notch institution, and align incentives all along the continuum to drive an acceptably cost-effective healthcare delivery system.

As the managed-care phenomenon has grown to gain the attention and favor of provider networks, we have not yet been able to lower our nation's overall costs. So what makes so many institutions, and so many physicians independent of their institutions, believe they can do better by direct contracting with employers or in some other way cutting the payor out of the loop? A crooked line of reasoning, mapping the new geography of healthcare coverage, drives this misguided thought process. The ambitious medical group wrongly assumes that a savvy provider can become a savvy payor simply by capturing the local population it already serves.

Managed care is all about serving populations not land areas. Employers and government agencies contract with managed-care organizations to deliver healthcare to their members, whenever and wherever they might need care. No matter whether you practice in a one-hospital town or in a strictly confined urban setting, where you may indeed control market share, invariably a certain amount of covered healthcare services must be delivered by providers located closer to members who frequently travel or live full-time outside of any definable zone. Quite often such out-of-area care delivery involves the most catastrophic and costly cases.

And it seems our nation's managed-care populations scatter a little farther afield every day. As more managed-care Medicare products arrive on the marketplace, for instance, we can expect a natural migration of a good many managed-care senior populations away from their home states for weeks, months, or years at a time. The story is much the same at the opposite end of the age curve. Children gone away to college and dependents living outside of the traditional family unit are members in good standing, too, although they cannot always be served by the local providers under their parents' or guardians' health plans.

Look again if you are convinced that such covered subpopulations constitute a small number. Out-of-area cases will likely have a major impact on your bottom line as the market moves from managed-care lite to heavy.

Costs, Outcomes, and Protocols First

Did someone say bottom line? That is getting ahead of the root problem, I would say. When it comes to measuring the cost of healthcare delivery and studying the human outcomes of clinical practice, neither bricks-and-mortar institutions nor large physician groups have a firm grip on the reality of their own organizations and marketplaces. Yet group after group declares its eagerness to tweak the raw numbers no one has gathered or analyzed in the first place and take on a serious new risk it little understands. Once again, the siren call of managed care's latest "thing to do" proves almost irresistible, and too many ill-prepared groups could wreck on that craggy shore.

Will medical groups eventually acquire the analytical acumen and administrative manpower to track and serve such far-flung populations most effectively? Possibly. But we are about ten years away from even satisfying the prerequisite course for such a scheme. Direct contracting will remain a foolhardy notion until the day some rationally organized provider system can actually digest and metabolize its own outcomes data and can get physicians agreeing to follow treatment protocols driven by those data.

Save a handful of extremely rare and dangerously alluring exceptions, I do not think any provider institution or physician group has demonstrated the lasting ability to contract directly with major employers.

PAYOR STRATEGIES

As we turn our attention to the third blade of the managed-care pinwheel, what most interests me is that today's managed-care payors, including those with a strong "national presence," are every bit as regionalized as the provider institutions and physician groups. All healthcare must be delivered locally, even by a plan that may rightfully claim interplanetary coverage and have its corporate headquarters situated as far away as Minnesota, Southern California, or Pennsylvania. As a matter of fact, the largest managed-care companies have been the least able to migrate their own best practices from one regional market to another.

Manage What Needs Managing

You see, most so-called managed-care payors have not been managing the healthy lives of their members but, rather, have been managing some financial aspects of the care system. Like the physicians and the institutions, these payor organizations have no understandable outcomes measures to describe their memberships, though they might know precisely how a certain financial incentive has reduced overall utilization.

With all the excess capacity remaining in the system, payors have been able to use classic supply/demand pressure to bring prices down among their suppliers, just as employers have used the same pressure to bring down premiums among payors in the emerging managed-care markets. In their desire to gain market share rapidly, beginning the moment they break into a new market, payors will take great pains to assemble the largest panel of physicians and hospitals possible.

In some instances, largely due to the providers' relative lack of sophisticated negotiation techniques, payors have been able to gain the earlier financial advantage by off-loading capitation risk onto providers. Though according to our index, provider acceptance of capitation risk indicates a managed-care heavy market, indeed such payors are really just squeezing managed-care lite markets. For providers who take the lead and accept those capitated risks contracts too early, the common problem is that the medical-loss ratios are set at too low a rate. So now the young plan has a broad panel, which is fantastic for marketing, but it wields little control over that panel, which undercuts the nobler causes of truly managing care or building any kind of understanding of health versus sickness across the network.

Eyes on the Index: Trimming the Panels

Here managed-care indexing holds great promise for a most practical application. As a marketplace emerges from a managed-care lite and into a managed-care heavy environment, the managed-care index can help a health plan know when best to prune its panel size. An informed plan can then assemble the tools it needs to zero in on meeting its population's needs, across the entire virtual geography of its marketplace. Specifically, the plan can begin by (1) laser targeting where its enrollees live and (2) custom tailoring its primary-care network around the actual travel times and shifting locations of members in its major employer groups. A plan situated in a market whose index score signals a rapid maturation can move with swiftness and confidence to trim its panel in the specialty arena. In time the plan might altogether drop specialists' names from its provider network listings, as the better part of the membership grows accustomed to following primary-care physicians' referrals with little or no question.

As its panel becomes more and more concentrated and its members are successfully channeled toward the very most appropriate physicians, a managed-care plan can stop worrying about restricting primary and specialty care and start targeting the overutilization of bricks-and-mortar resources. In all likelihood, tomorrow's thriving provider institutions will be the ones who have managed to establish the broadest continuums of service with the leanest assets and resources, a complex equation that must be balanced to help insurance companies control medical loss ratios. Flagship institutions, or institutions that fancy themselves flagships, are necessary in the beginning of a managed-care lite market but become less and less necessary as the market advances. A flagship at anchor can prove especially vulnerable to attack in a hotly competitive market, where members may be more willing to accept longer travel times.

The Fully Informed Payor

So for payors on the move from managed-care lite to managed-care heavy, a thoughtful interpretation of the managed-care index can help cultivate a deeper understanding of the real drivers of change in the marketplace. The payor armed with such an understanding is better able to navigate the ins and outs of provider contracting, to manage the care of its far-flung membership populations across suitably expansive geographic areas, and to craft its marketing campaigns to custom fit its panel or vice versa.

In other words, the index-smart payor is better equipped to manage its own business and business risks. Not that the formidable changes or challenges will cease, mind you. Accepting the risk of reimbursing reliable providers for care actually rendered versus prepaying a fixed amount per episode, presents another fundamentally new challenge for the payor that has worked so hard at off-loading such risk and has just nicely started cutting its roster of eligible physicians and facilities.

Often the provider institution believes that transferring its cost structure to business lines that are not initially controlled under contract by the payor will somehow give the provider a long-term strategic advantage. In reality, astute payor organizations are starting to acknowledge that they will have brighter prospects for lowering overall costs by sometimes contracting outside the traditional lines of business.

Payors are enjoying a newfound ability, for example to control drug costs not only via restricted drug formularies, but also through the pre-certification of pharmacies. As they follow the shift from lite to heavy managed-care market concentrations, payors find they can amass far greater buying power and soon shift their attention away from streamlining primary and specialty physician networks, and start nibbling away at the ancillary costs that can help them bring down their overall medical loss ratios faster still. That is why so many payors in advanced markets are scrambling to subcontract or "microcapitate" their alternative-setting offerings, such as mental health, rehabilitative, and long-term care.

S U M M A R Y

Putting the index to good work, in short, means putting the pinwheel to creative use. Again, the appropriate goal is not to outwit your partners in other sectors of the industry but, rather, to orchestrate a meeting of minds and a symphony of comprehensive, coordinated, cost-effective healthcare services across the community and, sometimes, beyond the immediate vicinity.

Providers that can offer "one-stop" contracting for the whole range of facility-based services, and medical groups that can provide similar convenience and efficiency in terms of guiding member populations from ancillary caregivers up through intensive care superspecialists, will enjoy a distinct advantage in tomorrow's managed-care marketplace. The ability to deliver fully comprehensive, easily accessible care will become increasingly important as we see point-of-service products entering managed-care heavy markets at a rapid rate, most notably becoming the product of choice for an exploding population of Medicare risk enrollees.

Among payors who refuse to migrate stepwise, from an indemnity thought process to a true managed-care process, a number of odd behaviors arise as the market advances. Too often I see indemnity insurance companies making awkward gestures toward a managed-care philosophy, usually by trying to cut and paste traditional indemnity systems, utilization techniques, and support functions onto a new so-called HMO or PPO product. The resulting Frankenstein's monster may at first glance appear cost-effective, but a closer examination reveals a body fashioned to resemble a managed-care organization controlled by a brain programmed to manipulate financial spreadsheets rather than manage the health of a human population. Even in extremely sophisticated managed-care markets one finds payors that, having made the transition to truly managing health, squander their hard-won success by getting into Medicare and Medicaid product lines and straining the same old systems and philosophies they use for their traditional commercial policyholders.

Experience tells me that, as the managed-care market becomes more sophisticated and more varied in its product offerings, the payor has to become practically schizophrenic in its strategic approach, setting up perhaps several products that may share some systems but essentially must stand alone in terms of marketing, membership services, and contracts.

To be successful in the Medicare market, for instance, one would do much better to set up what might be called an "HMO-within-an-HMO." Surely the unique needs of seniors call for a distinct HMO product, so that people can focus on the unique aspects of the Medicare recipient population and its unique healthcare continuum. Why dilute such a special population into the general membership?

Good managed care begins with a deep knowledge of the covered population and then follows through with decisive healthcare preventions and interventions based on that knowledge. A Medicare managed-care product should differ significantly from a commercial product in virtually every facet of its operations, from how memberships are sold to how care is delivered and providers contracted. And the same goes for products tailored for any of the other various subpopulations who constitute a health plan's valued membership. An index, a pinwheel, and a plan that does not work for people, does not work.

8
CHAPTER

Managing Organizational Change

Never before have strategic clairvoyance and operational flexibility been so critical to the future success of healthcare institutions and, indeed, of our entire industry. We need to know what is going to happen in the market before it happens, plot the surest course to a secure future, then act decisively without any serious missteps, to transform the key processes by which people, information, and technology combine to deliver just the right care at a superior value. Clearly such ambitious plans and actions are more handily managed at the micro than at the macro level. So our most influential architects of change may not be working on grand designs but rather on the smaller-scale redesign of everyday operations and strategies at their own institutions.

The present competitive environment only compounds a perennial challenge. Leveraged buyouts, mergers, acquisitions, and divestitures, Is this pinwheel of a market spinning too fast for the embattled institutional planner to grab hold? If we were not so fully occupied in charting the meteoric course, speed, and likely impact of such momentous change, some say, we might see the utter madness in it.

Fortunately, there is a proven method for dealing with this madness, change management. Whole shelves full of books have been published on the subject and standing armies of consultants deployed in the cause, yet change management is poorly understood and still more poorly practiced in healthcare today. Our aim here cannot be to exhaust this complex topic or even to provide an adequate crash course; it falls upon other dedicated publications and professional advisors to give change management the space and time it so richly deserves.

For the purposes of our argument, change management figures prominently as a fundamental managed-care technique and as an instrumental tool for piloting your organization's managed-care transformation. In this chapter we touch upon the guiding principles of change management, principles that managed-care organizations might wisely heed if they wish to survive and prosper as their market indexes rise.

A FEW CHANGE MANAGEMENT BASICS

The transformation of a managed-care marketplace and of its constituent provider, physician, and payor organizations cannot be accomplished without concerted effort and considerable pain. Even after having put forth the effort and endured pain, a lasting success may remain elusive. Some organizations just will not be equal to the task; their fate will be sealed soon enough. And not everyone who faithfully embarks upon the organizational change journey in a managed-care lite market will still be on board when the organization arrives in a managed-care heavy market. Heads will roll.

Healthcare organizational leaders need to face impending change and respond rationally and soberly with all the discipline they can muster. Gone are the days when leaders could mull over the future and casually discuss tomorrow's possibilities with their peers. The surviving players will be the ones who act, innovate, and stare down the stark truth that healthcare's classic institutions and honored traditions rest on shifting sand.

In particular, achieving success in change management means providing nimble leadership, knowing your target market and how to penetrate it, recognizing and rewarding value, constantly learning and retooling, forging mutually advantageous alliances, rendering second-to-none service to all users, and rapidly adapting to changing market conditions. It is quite a juggling act. Most of all, though, the success of any change process rests upon the shoulders of the very people who will be paving the way or following an inspiring lead.

Leadership

One prediction you can bank on is that the fierce competitive pressures in today's healthcare market will persist for years to come, reinforcing the "more-for-less" campaigns that first sparked the managed-care movement and now continue to fuel the present revolution. In a heated market that will demand more output from everyone, while offering fewer assurable personal rewards, healthcare leaders must find a way to work collaboratively with the various constituents who follow their cues.

Leaders must empower their followers, as followers must accept more responsibility for work outcomes. Specifically, the new working relationship must be founded on leaders' effective delegation of responsibility for planning and control, absolutely critical activities in any changing environment.

Team Building

Given the inescapable premise that, in the healthcare workforce of the future, people at all levels will have much more autonomy and control over their work, the assembly of multidisciplinary, cross-functional teams is looking like a more and more attractive alternative to the traditional wire-diagram organizational chart, with its one big box at the top supported by a human pyramid of subordinate boxes. Instead, organizations should be structured more creatively, so people can achieve the best use of their skills and accomplish tasks in ways that make the most sense in performing the work.

Teamwork and efficiency do not just sprout organically from a leader's irresistible force of will. The successful team must be built with dedicated members who are:

- Carefully selected;
- Expertly trained;
- Adequately rewarded for the value they add; and
- Assured job security and ample opportunity for advancement.

Integrate all these basic components into your team concept and great things will happen; leave any one component out and team building quickly becomes just another fruitless exercise, a reshuffling of names in the same old hat.

Reward and Recognition

Nothing less than a revolution is under way in the field of personnel management. Employers in healthcare and elsewhere are discarding the time-honored merit pay system, under which employees in the American workplace have long been rewarded according to fixed promotion schedules and pay scales.

Value-based compensation is the name of the game today. More employers are setting up systems by which they can gauge a person's competitive market value in a specific geographic area then "incentivize" the job to reap that value. Incentives are geared toward securing an employee's or physician's promised or potential value added, and rewards fluctuate from year to year depending on the individual's actual contribution to the organization's overall performance, whether financial or strategic. Value-based incentives might extend to entire workgroups in a team setting.

Such constant reward and recognition of valuable work accomplishments is an essential component of any effort to manage change. Vigorous change is best carried out by vigorously motivated people, after all. So today's astute leaders are busy operationalizing the widely demonstrated power of nonfinancial (intrinsic) rewards to motivate and sustain superior employee performance. Daily, these innovators prove that the best employees or physicians, whether leaders or followers, appreciate being recognized for a quality job well done.

Technology and Training

Considering the unprecedented pace and sweep of change in the healthcare marketplace today, training all personnel to keep up with or get ahead of advancements in their respective fields has become an absolutely essential component of sound organizational management. Training should be focused on fundamental behavioral and technical skills as well as on the unique competencies required of the various leaders and followers in your organization.

Change management ties every training program to the organization's broader strategic objectives and business goals. Every year or so, an organization should reassess its human-skill base and ensure that base provides the desirable competitive edge.

Strategic and Tactical Planning

In such a swiftly moving and highly competitive market, today's health-care organization can no longer afford to shoot from the hip when making major business decisions. Rather, executive decisions, and even the most basic managerial actions, must be based on an intimate knowledge of the organization's overall business direction. Only a carefully designed and fully understood business strategy will keep leaders from getting distracted and wasting time on wholly inappropriate activities. Cultivating the discipline to improve constantly, keeping one eye always on the pinwheel, and sticking to your knitting will be the essential ingredient of organizational survival and success in tomorrow's managed-care environment.

ASSEMBLING THE CHANGE MANAGEMENT TEAM

Throughout the 27 years of my career in healthcare management, I have witnessed or "midwifed" an extraordinary number of change processes with some successes, some noble attempts, and some utter but highly educational failures. Most of the time, it seems, I must begin such engagements by talking the executives down from a precarious height. The leaders of healthcare institutions are wont to get the entire organization involved, as if the broadest possible involvement, in and of itself, will create the required momentum for change.

Nothing could be further from the truth. Of the several hundreds of volumes on change management now in print, none puts broad participation anywhere near strong leadership on the list of critical success factors. My consulting experience bears this out. Only executive leaders can take the bold, practical steps I have seen work at healthcare organizations that have successfully acknowledged the need to change, created the wherewithal to change, and actually effected some positive change.

The Chief Executive Officer

Only the Chief Executive Officer (CEO) can lead the change campaign. This is my first sacred principle of change management. The role of a manager, vice-president, or senior vice-president who first sees a need for change is to convince the chief executive to lead the pursuit. The CEO has to act not only as the champion of change, but also as one who will be intimately involved in working toward the institution's new direction.

Looking once again to the pinwheel, we can better understand that perhaps the greatest challenge for today's chief executives lies in creating new and different relationships among payors, bricks-and-mortar provider organizations, or physician groups. For too long these market sectors have been downright hostile toward one another or, at best, not very trusting. How frequently these days we hear news about failed joint ventures and their failed struggles to make change management work. Total Quality Management, Visioning, Management by Objectives, Zero-based Budgeting, or whatever name it might go by, your average change management initiative flashes across the monitor faster than last quarter's financial results.

Forging the new relationships that might give change management a fighting chance in today's marketplace will be no cinch. CEOs are navigating in uncharted waters with little or no guidance, other than the knowledge they may have gathered from the many previous models that failed. But remember, failure can be our best teacher.

The Office of Managed-Care Development

For any player on either blade of the pinwheel, whether an indemnity insurance company, a physician group, or a healthcare institution moving confidently from a managed-care lite to a managed-care heavy market will require an unprecedented concentration of will and a focus of effort. Such a transformation is best managed from within by a multidisciplinary team assembled under a confident leader. The resulting Office of Managed-Care Development, as I and my clients most often call it, directs the partnerships and innovations that, over time will distinguish the organization as a sophisticated managed-care provider.

At the helm of the Office of Managed-Care Development should be one dedicated professional who is solely responsible for using the managed-care index to monitor your organization's progress and who is eminently capable of motivating your institution, physician group, or insurance company to acquire and refine the managed-care techniques that will shape your healthcare market.

A carefully staffed Office of Managed-Care Development, led by such a professional or managed-care "czar," must then be freed to spend the time it takes to act upon and react to the various contracts the institution or the provider panel sign. More important, the Office must be authorized to implement the information and care delivery systems that will facilitate the most cost-effective operations and the most favorable return on the organization's investment in managed care.

In short, the Office of Managed-Care Development should become your organization's new headquarters for success in a changing healthcare market. One could just as well call it the Office of Managed-Care Enlightenment. The learning managed-care organization moves beyond a philosophy that asks "How do we get enough covered lives so we will not have to change anything we do?" to a philosophy that asks "Once we capture our market share, which may never amount to more than 30 percent of covered lives in this market, how can we survive or even prosper?" An invaluable resource to executive leaders and all constituents of the change management campaign, the Office of Managed-Care Development asks the right strategic questions then helps formulate and operationalize the right answers.

The Board of Directors

As the wider marketplace grows to recognize that managing care means much more than merely managing finances (more in Chapter 9), and as long as we still have excess capacity in our healthcare delivery system, many institutions are going to be called upon to actually eliminate themselves or change beyond recognition. Many of these institutions may boast a proud history of community service and dedication to healing; their losses, though assuredly necessary, will be sad and sometimes hurtful. Unlike the so-called market consolidations of the recent past, this next wave of consolidations and closings will actually reduce capacity by eliminating the obvious excesses, especially in terms of inpatient beds. The industry cannot abide another flurry of net inactivity, in which a few organizations simply change their names from hospital to medical center or from PPO to HMO.

Closures, sales, mergers, and other drastic measures call for sure-footed leadership, of course, as well as informed governance. The enlightened CEO who is able to convince the Board of Directors of the wisdom of his or her strategy must then count the votes closely, probably several times. It is always better to have the Board on your side, fully informed, and with a clear vision of the strategy you are about to undertake, even if it takes several months to achieve consensus.

Members of the Board must also be made to understand the dynamics of today's burgeoning managed-care marketplace. Remember that your institution is not seeking to win at the expense of another institution along the traditional continuum of care but, rather, to cultivate partnerships with all three components of your own pinwheel in order to beat out or absorb other pinwheels across the market. Board members who wince at the very mention of the word "competition" might well be comforted by such an insight.

Inertia is another fundamental principle of change that chief executives and Boards must acknowledge and obey. As a clever planner once asked me, "Why is it we never have time to plan it right, but we always have time to redo it later?" Because once you begin the change process, I replied, it quickly builds up too great a momentum for you to stop and start again. Stutter-starting will not only kill the change process, it will likely also sacrifice the job of the person who started the change and started the process in motion.

Yet another change principle falls under the category of "loose lips sink ships." The heady liquor of the grapevine brims to overflowing in times of turmoil. And the Board members are the ones who will get wind of all the juiciest misinformation first. Clear, frequent, and honest communication between the CEO and the Board is the only preemptive strike that can win the inevitable war of words.

The Management Team

Moving in parallel with an enlightened chief executive and an informed Board, the Management Team, must transform itself into a lean and nimble body. First of all, people are going to have to migrate from a departmental to a system focus, because in managed care everything is a cost center. It does not matter whether you are the insurer tackling general and administrative expenses, the physician provider tackling care delivery and claims processes, or the bricks-and-mortar administrator tackling the average daily census. You must constantly be challenging yourself and everyone with whom you interact to ascertain whether another part of the pinwheel can do the job better, faster, and with higher quality while lowering cost and improving the health of the population you jointly serve.

In other words, your management team cannot be blinded by its history or contained by the traditional four walls of the institution. Instead, tomorrow's effective managers must restlessly seek every possibly better methodology to cut costs, transfer medical delivery to more appropriate settings, and move away from a sickness to a population health concern, all while remaining financially viable or, better yet, improving financial performance.

Cross-Organizational Teams

The boundary walls start crumbling as a market emerges into a managed-care heavy environment and the pinwheels start forming. Once your own institutions' management teams buy in to the change process, executive leaders will need to create cross-organizational teams to tend the pinwheel and the systemwide issues that might otherwise fall between the cracks.

As the market shifts its focus away from worrying about who gets what part of the premium dollar and toward determining the most appropriate use of that premium dollar, management must begin to plan care processes and the delivery of population healthcare between formerly competing, and sometimes combative entities. Considering the breadth of such an enterprise, only a pinwheel-wide cooperative of insurance executives, physician executives, hospital, ambulatory care, long-term care, home health, and other professionals can realistically organize and manage it. The various members of this cross-organizational team must sit together as equals, instead of bickering about who is the first-, second-, or third-class citizen across the table.

Cross-organizational managers will have to delegate their day-to-day operational responsibilities to other departmental leaders, so they can spend time outside the four walls. There simply are not enough hours in a day to manage both institutional and extra-institutional matters. A cross-organizational management team will have to be constantly scanning the population horizon to both see things and be seen as a community player. It will no longer be enough to sign a contract and leave it cast in stone until the next contract opening. The fabric of the pinwheel will need constant mending.

MANAGING INTERINSTITUTIONAL AND COMMUNITY CHANGE

Over time, through numerous trials and tribulations, the cross-institutional teaming will also dictate how many organizations can comfortably and effectively relate to each other. A good pinwheel holds only so many entities. In today's more successfully integrated mature markets, only a handful of pinwheels interact. As long as they are constantly lowering costs and improving health for those that they serve, a few players can dominate a market for some time. Market dominance will be a function of a pinwheel's ability to constantly rightsize, cooperate, learn, and improve.

Overcapacity lingers like a big headache for interinstitutional managers. Through mergers and acquisitions, more and more excess capacity will have to be removed from our healthcare system. Eventually, as pinwheels upon pinwheels form, spin off, and reform, a few will achieve dominance, begin truly competing, and wield their sheer market force to milk the last remnants of overcapacity out of the system. Needless to say, a few brave leaders are going to have to volunteer for the toughest mission and that is to stay behind the advancing front, quietly turn off the lights, and lock the doors. Again, these leaders must find solace in the knowledge that their sacrifice will improve the health of their community and reduce the exorbitant cost of care.

Inside the institution, we will see a lot less of the absurd hierarchy and fragmentation that has plagued our system and a lot more collaboration and interaction around clinical processes. Still, the more prevalent trend will be the expansion of these clinical processes beyond the four walls that any one institution owns.

Some, but not many, healthcare organizations have already embarked upon this change process. Traditional suppliers of drugs, for example, are no longer justifying their costs based simply on clinical superiority but, more to the point, on how their products affect the total cost of care and, ultimately, the well-being of the individual. The seemingly divergent goals of better health and lower costs, these manufacturers are beginning to see, cannot so easily be separated. Drug distribution systems are also being tailored for the new managed-care reality. Maintenance drugs can now be ordered and delivered by mail to a member's doorsteps, much more effectively maintaining a member's health while significantly lowering our overall cost.

For the professional provider, such innovations at the interinstitutional and community level sound a fanfare for real change. So many of the time-honored and facility-bound aspects of our care delivery system were developed and have been long maintained for the system's own convenience. We are fortunate indeed to be watching that system flex and strain to provide superior convenience for those who most deserve it: our paying plan members and, in time, the population as a whole.

SUMMARY

A new millennium looms just over the horizon, and so the sun is rising on a new era in healthcare. Our industry's ablest organizations are acting now to seize this moment of opportunity. Slow movers, one might reasonably conclude, may soon be doomed to the scrap heap.

Not only is change unpleasant, but it takes a long, long time. If you find the change process delightful and swift, you are doing it all wrong. But once a chief executive officer sees the need for change and commits his or her core leaders to the journey, positive change can happen in due course. Strong leadership will make all the difference in the world. Today's astute healthcare executive already has assembled innovative and strong-willed team leaders who have the courage to risk failure, laugh in the face of uncertainty, and remain focused but flexible.

These leaders in turn have attracted followers who are more than eager to work in a fast-moving environment that will tap every ounce of knowledge, skill, and talent one has to offer. Such teams do not merely grasp opportunity, they create it themselves. And this wonderfully collaborative relationship between leaders and followers enables an organization to hone its skills and step up to competitors whenever market forces dictate.

Once the change management revolution reaches a fever pitch, we are going to start to see reward systems tied not only to organizational objectives, but to community health objectives as well. Whatever health and financial outcomes we endeavor to measure and reward should be ripe with new opportunities to change behaviors for the better.

Consider the insurance executive who elevates the health of the served population and lowers primary-care costs by drafting a creative contract with a wellness center, including aroma therapy, thus lowering the premium while maintaining his bottom line. Consider the system executive who, through a combination of owning and contracting, takes on full risk for a continuum of care, enabling her to close half the hospital beds while reducing the percent of premium needed for the institutional component of the medical loss ratio. Finally, consider the group of primary-care physicians who cut back on mental health referrals by hiring a full-time psychologist as a physician extender.

Anyone who cannot see what exciting, changing times we live in must be Walt Disney's cryogenic bunkmate. With so many of American healthcare's traditional platforms now burning, and so many complicating and unstabilizing forces threatening to hurl the market into chaos, when will today's conscientious executive leaders ever find the time to pause, take one step back, and enjoy a leisurely look at where their organizations should be heading? Not in our lifetime; not if leaders fail to cultivate the vital discipline by which long-range visioning and short-term change processes are harnessed together.

Such a living discipline of organizational planning and change management must become a matter of top priority rather than an exercise designed to occupy spare time. The stakes are just too high for us to commit to anything less than the wholehearted management of organizational change, from institution to institution, pinwheel to pinwheel, to all across this industry.

9

CHAPTER

After the Revolution

Recent trends and current actions that I observe in today's most mature managed-care marketplaces give me ample reason to hope that, against all odds and contrary to public opinion, American healthcare might be moving in the right direction after all. Together we are striving to construct an equitable financing and delivery model, bearing at least a striking resemblance to my managed-care pinwheel, by which the healthcare industry can someday accomplish the truly free exchange of intellectual capital by which our society can modestly approach a system of total population health management.

Look at the very hub of the pinwheel. Consider the latest breakthroughs in the development and practical application of both advanced information technologies and effective case management techniques, the linchpins of tomorrow's virtually integrated delivery systems. We are in the midst of a veritable information renaissance, bringing bright new hopes that we can soon establish vital information system connectivity and data repositories, such as electronic community health records, which must pave the way for the sharing of intellectual capital. And with the refinement and proliferation of powerful new case management techniques, tomorrow's payors, providers, and physicians can work to catapult their shared intellectual capital into more intelligent preventions, interventions, and care processes, all with a sharp eye toward better health outcomes for their member populations.

So most of the pieces seem to be falling into place, at long last, and most of the players are finding their chairs. So are we glimpsing the beginning of an end, already, to this young market revolution? Not a chance. Any useful model of the future must keep spinning forward, in living motion, propelled by the ever-changing needs and preferences of healthcare consumers and by the ever-increasing ability of payors, physicians, and providers to manage health, not just finances.

THE NEW HEALTHCARE CONSUMERISM

The managed-care industry has been boasting health management successes it may have a hard time documenting, and enthusiastic champions like me have been extending other promises that insurers, doctors, and hospitals may have an even harder time keeping. Plan members and potential new enrollees have been listening and have come to expect the utmost in service and quality. We all demand a better value for our healthcare dollar these days.

Enter a strong new wave of healthcare consumerism. This inertial movement is perhaps best exemplified by the growing popularity of point-of-service plans, which allow members to go outside the closed HMO network of doctors and hospitals in exchange for a slightly higher premium and copayment. Point-of-service products may finally succeed in attracting those vast multitudes who, wanting not to forfeit any personal choice at any price, have been sorely reluctant to enroll in managed-care plans.

Still, the mounting healthcare consumer movement goes far beyond a demand for more freedom of choice at the point of service.

A Clamor for Reliable Information

Whether understanding or misunderstanding their supposed power to select their own practitioners and to control their own care processes, healthcare consumers now crave the basic information they need to best exercise these newfound powers. The media are more than glad to feed people's hunger for reliable, thoughtful health information. Some journalists have risen to the challenge most admirably. The best and most eagerly devoured reports go beyond the usual self-care and screening tips or hollow advice to seek professional help, one can now learn a surprising lot from books, magazines, newspapers, and television about how to use our changing healthcare system. And that is the kind of guidance today's consumer can really use.

A recent special pullout in the Wall Street Journal* for example, came packed with brief but cogent how-to articles, geared to the curious and sophisticated healthcare consumer. Assuming that readers had some knowledge of current marketplace events, but never glossing over the fundamentals, the publication dispensed friendly advice on selecting an HMO, choosing a physician, assembling the right benefits package, saving on drug costs, better medical financial planning through flexible "medspend" accounts, appealing a rejected claim, gauging the worth of provider report cards, and even deciphering a laboratory's biopsy analysis.

Such responsibly thorough and insightful news coverage, in fact, has become commonplace in the press and on television. Even if a feature story in the local newspaper or on television provides skimpy facts and gives consumers nothing more than a morsel of food for thought, the reporter's heart is usually in the right place. And readers', listeners', and viewers' need for solid information stands at an all-time high. More than ever before, patients in the managed-care era must be informed and participative in their own care. A massive consumer movement could do the cause a world of good right about now.

A sound managed-care plan requires a robust educational component, not only to achieve superior prevention, self-care, screening, and clinical management, but also to tell curious consumers how best to use a financing and delivery system that many are still unfamiliar. The media, so often tagged as enemies of the managed-care revolution, can be invaluable partners in this regard and should be encouraged to perform a vital public service.

The Paradox of Choice

Informed choice and participation in care are desirable ideals for our emerging healthcare system, we all agree. But as healthcare consumers grow more and more savvy, they too will realize that, as a society, our greatest opportunity to achieve real value lies in the superior management of population health. Too much insistence on choice may be the most se-

---

*("Surviving the Squeeze: A Guide to Stretching Your Healthcare Dollar," special Section R, 24 Oct 1996)

rious threat to the manageable, economically responsible system of public health I envision.

We are not even close to fulfilling the greatest promise of the managed-care revolution, and we might never get there unless we can strike some rather painful but, I believe, quite necessary compromises in the years ahead. In this need for compromise lies a not-so-subtle paradox. Each of us must give up some dearly held power or freedom in order to empower every citizen with the freedom to enjoy access to high-quality healthcare.

The managed-care pinwheel concept shows how the payor, physician group, and bricks-and-mortar sectors of the marketplace are regrouping to effectively abandon their cross-industry conquests. Today's leading market players realize that, to achieve their highest potential as business enterprises, they must give up the folly of owning and controlling other parts of the system.

Overall system value depends on the efficient operation of each industry segment, and a huge component of that efficiency lies in directing patients to the most appropriate providers and settings. So plan members must realize that they would do better, in the long run, to yield the power of choice in many instances. In the United States, where placing any limit on choice, however well intentioned or convincingly reasoned, such an utterance might be considered a criminal offense. Although nationwide enrollment in choice-limiting HMOs has skyrocketed, the trend will reach a natural end. True managed care, featuring certain limits on patient choice, will be a tough sale among people who can afford the luxury of total choice or who choose to risk carrying no health insurance whatsoever.

True, a few stubborn blocs of resistance could make it difficult or impossible for managed care to fulfill its highest aspirations for total population health management. Call it managed care's promised land; I may not get there with you. The important thing is to keep the vision in sight and, in the interim, to do our very best to fulfill managed care's shorter-term promise as a strictly members-only proposition. If the population of covered lives someday matches the population of the United States, fine; if not, we will still have come a long, long way in the right direction.

BEYOND MANAGED FINANCING

So far, the debate about managed care has really been a debate about managed financing. We have been far more concerned about cost than we have about quality or access, the other essential terms in the value equation. Are managed-care payors picking institutions based on price alone? The anecdotal evidence would seem to support that thesis. Is that any way to run a healthcare system?

But the business literature rarely, if ever, acknowledges that the lowest-cost institutions selected and used by managed-care companies operate the same old clinical programs they always have. Managed care today is hastily built on the smoking ruins of the fee-for-service industry. I have not stumbled across one exposé or scorecard report that truthfully characterizes the fee-for-service system as an insatiable monster that, for too long, has greedily ingested more of our gross domestic product than has any other healthcare system in any other civilized nation, without giving the United States an equivalent top-health ranking.

Nor do we hear often enough how a fee-for-service reimbursement scheme created a healthcare system that, through ever-increasing premiums, created an oversupply of medically trained personnel. People got licensed and performed various treatments without any oversight, as long as the license was kept up-to-date. "Choice at any cost" was the battle cry of the professionals who were only too happy to receive the ever higher fees. Unfortunately for these very professionals, who today are grabbing the short end of the managed-care stick, the benefits of choice did not pass along to the employers and governments who were footing the bill.

Is Bad Managed Care Better Than None At All?

Suddenly, out of nowhere, comes a concept of managed financing, cleverly disguised as managed care. But even this sham, as some would call it, or precursor of true managed care, I would call it, has easily outperformed the outmoded fee-for-service scheme.

Managed healthcare financing has succeeded in reducing premiums without causing any demonstrated adverse impact on the health of the nation, as best we can measure health in the general population. As a matter of fact, most of the objective studies show that managed financing, through incentives that at least pantomime the techniques of true managed care, has even improved the delivery of preventive care. The earlier intervention of qualified healthcare professionals is something the fee-for-service system neither encouraged nor denied but rarely paid for.

On the other hand, aggressive payor initiatives have had a significantly adverse impact on the incomes of physicians, hospitals, and the many professionals who work in hospitals and other healthcare organizations. Left unchecked, this disturbing trend in the healthcare economy might cause lasting damage.

How did we get here? Brushing up on their Adam Smith, the managed-care industry moguls applied the Theory of Supply and Demand to bargain their way into deep price discounts, based on the promise of higher volume for physicians and providers. Much to the discredit of the bona fide managed-care industry, especially payors, these discounts were falsely negotiated under the banner of health maintenance organizations. Maintaining health hardly crossed anyone's mind.

Now, and we should not be surprised, most physicians and most all of the American public view managed care in the wrong light. Many feel they have been sold a package labeled "managed care" only to unwrap it and find a product that manages everything but care. Insurers manage policyholders' choice of physician, access to providers, and claims approvals as well as doctors' referral processes and practice patterns. These payors claim to be lowering the cost of healthcare by improving the health of members, but rarely do they openly advertise that they are reaping most of their member savings and corporate profits through selected exclusions of benefits and volume discounts.

To picture the problem in cruder terms, think of our managed-care impostors as automobile manufacturers with unheard-of power in their marketplace. What if car makers advertised a luxury sedan that would cost no more to operate than an economy hatchback? But, to make good on their bold claim, designers need never bother to reengineer the sedan for greater fuel economy; instead, bargainers could just muscle the oil companies to slash the price of gasoline. Now the station attendant, the tanker trucker, the guy who owns ten stations in your city, and maybe even J. R. Ewing himself must suffer the consequences of the car manufacturers' good fortune.

With such imbalance in the broader marketplace, it cannot be long before the lucky drivers start suffering, too. Soon they might rather swap that cheap gas for a more plentiful supply and reliable, excellent service with a smile.

Eyes on the Road, Please

Managed care, as we know it today, needs a lot of work; managed care, as we will surely know it tomorrow, will take a lot of work, too. We are merely feeling the growing pains of managed care's long, hard adolescence.

But imagine the rich possibilities for the future. One bright idea has won the undivided attention of the whole healthcare industry. Unlike governmentally imposed reform, market self-reform cannot be shouted down or lobbied away. Even our most staunchly opposed professionals and administrators have come to recognize that, like it or not, the managed-care phenomenon is not going to go away. In fact, the reform movement grows stronger every day. Hospitals that only recently feared they would never earn their charges back are starting to talk about receiving a percentage of fixed and variable costs, and then reengineering to regain profitability. For the first time in the history of American healthcare, success is not strictly a function of what, where, or who your organization is, but a simple matter of what it can demonstrate and negotiate on the open market.

Much to its credit, the healthcare industry has done many things, most notably in the pioneer days of managed care, for the express purpose of improving the health of the populations for which it is responsible. Many of the trailblazers who entered the field early and nurtured their fledgling organizations from small group models to multistate health maintenance organizations all of a sudden faced a huge need for capital. To some, meeting that need for capital meant converting to a for-profit entity, which brought the additional discipline of economic return imposed by Wall Street, a concept of both health and economic value that had not been imposed on the not-for-profit entity.

Given this new market reality in healthcare, featuring open competition and close scrutiny by investors, many professionals who have not taken kindly to being in oversupply, and thus being forced to negotiate in a classic Adam Smith model, instead have taken the moral high ground. The hardcore zealots view any concern for the financial aspects of healthcare as unfeeling, at best, or unethical, at worst. This stance I find most peculiar, whether viewing the past, the present, or the future of healthcare. These moralists are the very professionals, after all, who have long caused the rising cost of medical care to far and away exceed the inflationary rate of the Consumer Price Index. They created a system that sorely needs fixing, they should be most interested in seeing that the job is done right, and they and their patients stand to gain as much as anybody under a system of true managed care. Flouting the prevailing winds of change is one thing, resisting change altogether is quite another.

The pressing need to add both economic and health value is the central issue of managed care, as this book has tried so hard to reiterate on page after page. Managed care does not equal managed financing. Managing care is all about knowing that a similar organization, at the same stage of market development, and facing a similar case was able to collect sound data, analyze it, negotiate payments around the full spectrum of necessary interventions, and actually try to influence the delivery of those interventions to improve the health of its members. Managed care is about professionals who, having been charged with full responsibility for the clinical care of a member population, are trying to understand and change interventions to be more cost-effective, while maintaining and even improving quality. Managed care is about institutions that once delivered care exclusively at the inpatient bedside and are now answering the challenge to seek the most appropriate alternative settings and entering true partnerships with their professional staffs to make the bold innovations such a profound transformation will require.

S U M M A R Y

I believe the healthcare debate, like this book, is moving into a new chapter. In the United States the debate has always revolved around the question, Who will finance care? The answer to that question grew painfully obvious as the federal reform movement fizzled. Healthcare will always be financed by many different sectors of our society. Every one of those sectors, all those who pay for healthcare, today demands a better economic value as well as a better health value for their hard-earned money.

Our best prospects for reaping value, and indeed for the future of health in America, rests in the hands of those managed-care organizations, be they payors, providers, or some yet unknown entities that can best demonstrate an understanding of the health status of their member populations as a whole, analyze various subpopulations' health needs in minutiae, then intervene clinically and sociologically to improve health. Such a system must constantly improve itself, as well, to reduce costs and to remove any barriers to the appropriate behaviors, actions, and lifestyles that create and maintain a healthy population.

Will any of our classic healthcare institutions, as we know them, survive the inferno of change? I believe not. But new organizations, like phoenixes, will arise out of the ashes. Already we are seeing new organizations enter partnerships that just a few years ago would have seemed impossible. New spins on old affiliations, payment methodologies, and corporate structures arise every day. I think we are starting to see good old-fashioned Yankee innovation enter the healthcare market and displace the feudal-guild system of healthcare delivery.

So after the revolution expect the next revolution. The resulting national healthcare system will be a vast network of regionally organized systems concerned with managing health. And managing "health," as the World Health Organization defines the term, means not only striving to wipe out disease, but also organizing precious resources to enhance the social and economic well-being of a population.

A F T E R W O R D

We are just nicely putting this book to bed as the hubbub of another election year begins, bringing virtually no change in our nation's executive or legislative leadership and no brilliant new ideas about how the government can really help improve American healthcare today and tomorrow. Needless to say, I did not stay up all night watching the vote tallies. For healthcare, the meaningful victories and concessions had been declared months and years before.

Candidates predictably will stick to the easy topics, incumbents straining to congratulate themselves for making benefits slightly more portable, and everyone sharing a cautionary word about gagging and binding physician gatekeepers, joining the surefire rants against preexisting conditions and "drive-by" (sic) deliveries, and scrapping to a "Mediscare" stalemate while nodding in general agreement that the program can and must be saved. All the humdrum orators were speechless whenever the opportunity arose to champion or attack the fundamental principles and shaping market forces explored in these pages.

Who can blame the ambitious politician and the wary spin doctor? What intelligent remark might one usefully add to a managed population healthcare movement-in-progress that has taken on such a rich life of its own? But a breezy campaign and a status-quo election result by no means signal a state of equilibrium in healthcare policy or in any national affairs, foreign or domestic. The name-calling spats and budget battles have not skipped a beat.

Besides, the political season in the past did bring constructive action and tidbits of heartening news on some local fronts. California voters, who know managed care better than most, defeated two propositions that called for tighter state control over HMOs. It seems the majority in my own home state still believes that, in a free market, your average managed-care organization can outperform any government agency in responding to consumers' real health needs and preferences. Somehow managed care was able to weather the tough rhetoric of its many outspoken opponents, including the sometimes unduly harsh critics in the press. Chalk this one up to the long experience of California's millions of HMO members, who generally have enjoyed excellent service, sound value, and consistently high satisfaction rates.

MIND THE MATTER

Veteran public servants and astute voters heed the clever adage: One may campaign in poetry but must govern in prose. Elected representatives do have their work cut out for them. Never before has there been such pressure to curb healthcare spending and get a handle on the runaway social endowments, Medicare and Medicaid.

Throughout this book I have been loath to cite the coldest of the innumerable cold statistics, but sometimes numbers do paint the clearest picture. According to the HCFA home page* the United States spent $51 billion on healthcare in 1967, or 6.3% of the Gross National Product. Total HCFA spending reached $248.9 billion, or 16.4% of the federal budget, in 1995. Federal healthcare expenditures per person have exploded from $247 in 1967 to a whopping $3510 by 1994.

The dollars speak volumes, but how do they figure? At this late date, does everyone not know that rising costs are not the country's root public health problem? Healthcare's economic woes are merely a symptom of an underlying disease state, and it is a *social* disease. The demographic tidal wave of our nation's rapidly aging population has not even crested yet, and the chasm between our society's haves and have-nots just grows wider and deeper with each passing year. The population covered by Medicare has nearly doubled since the program's inception, from 19.5 million in 1967 to a projected 38.1 million in 1996. Likewise, the fifty states' Medicaid rolls have grown steadily in the present decade; program recipients constituted 10.2% of the total civilian population in 1990 and 13.8% in 1996, for an increase exceeding 35%.

Government officials should resist the urge to tamper with regulation and policy details and instead concern themselves with the gargantuan task of shoring up the United States' crumbling social infrastructure. After all, an effective healthcare financing and delivery system, public or private, can only be built on the very firmest of foundations. We face the very same socioeconomic challenge, I hasten to add, in managing welfare, education, and so many other essential components of the national life.

MIND THE BACKLASH

Let our other great social institutions take care of our great societal ills. When it comes to demonstrating value, the healthcare industry must fend

---

*Based on a report from the Bureau of Data Management, "1996 HCFA Statistics," HCFA Publication No. 03394, September 1996.

for itself. But even in the face of such formidable economic challenges, too many healthcare industry leaders have demonstrated reluctance to embrace proven economic solutions. Managed care still suffers from a pervasive fear that Big Business and healthcare make strange bedfellows. In today's burgeoning managed-care environment, the Flat Earth Societies boast record memberships. Where most observers foresee sure progress, some are just as sure to find roiling uncertainty and danger.

If Medicare was our industry's moonshot and Prospective Payment its Shuttle program, then managed care is a permanently manned, privately funded space colony. On the flip side of that commemorative medallion, of course, the more cynical reader glosses another inscription: If Medicare was our *Apollo 13* and Prospective Payment our *Challenger* disaster, then managed care is a full-scale Martian invasion. Of course the diehard skeptics are never at a loss for excuses. Some will clutch any current event, from the newest strain of computer virus to alleged fraud in the Human Genome Project, as proof enough the sky is falling. Ever since Kitty Hawk they have been bellyaching that man was never meant to fly.

Not a day goes by, it seems, without yet another high-profile report about some medical calamity, no doubt solely attributable to an evil cabal of managed-care profiteers. We Americans do so love a conspiracy theory. One recent study* confirms my suspicion that negative stories about managed care outnumber positive stories five to one. Popular targets range from denial of care and "drive-through" deliveries to executive compensations and physician "gag orders."

We need strong antidotes for such anecdotes. How many more medical calamities are being averted every day by refreshingly preventive efforts involving superior member education, screening, self-care, followup, and case management under true managed care plans? And how many of the most widely publicized horror stories involve the Indemnity-in-Drag plans that are managed care in name only? The occasional Public Relations setback should not faze our master planning or sap our confidence. Armed with equally compelling *positive* stories, we must frequently and calmly profess our knowledge that, on the whole, managed care is the best, not perfect, financing and delivery mechanism for the next American century.

Having presumably read the preceding chapters, you know that strong-arm gatekeepers, knee-jerk denials of care, and jackbooted discharges have no place in the brave new managed care world I envision.

---

*Reported in the 4 November 1996 issue of *Modern Healthcare,* "Survey confirms HMOs' bad press," p. 10.

Honing basic managed-care techniques that obviate the need for these intolerable practices will be a much easier and less disruptive task if we focus all eyes always on the higher principles. We must determine which practices have been part of the problem and which ones must be part of tomorrow's healthcare solution. Nor should we tolerate the notion that certain human casualties are to be expected and accepted as the natural costs of our long transition to managed care. No destination, however beckoning, is worth going down that trail of tears. We need leave no one behind.

A number of respected authors, most recently the *Wall Street Journal's* George Anders in *Health Against Wealth: HMOs and the Breakdown of Medical Trust* (Houghton Mifflin, 1996), back the managed-care backlash with a thoroughness and intelligence that cannot easily be dismissed. Again, the examples they cite usually recount practices that have no place in true managed care. Most bemoan the cold-hearted industrialization of American medicine, where the fatigued caregiving team forms a thoughtless unit of production and the unfortunate patients serve as their cheap, interchangeable parts. But, tell me, what makes the managed care plan so much colder and more calculating than healthcare businesses of the past? How soon we forget the impersonal bedside manners of the quasi-military bureaucracies, clerical hierarchies, and amateur administrations that have dominated healthcare for so many generations.

Ours is a curiously modern predicament, with deep roots in the early twentieth-century mind. "Things fall apart," goes this particular brand of apocalyptic noodling, "The centre cannot hold. Mere anarchy is loosed upon the world." The population explosion is having its way with us. Healthcare and other established institutions of the public trust must confront a brand-new reality every five or ten years. Indeed we are witnessing the death struggle of our classic healthcare institutions and should not be surprised if the drama is gripping, the players intense, and the soundtrack positively operatic! But to divide the healthcare stage, with good doctors and patients on one side against evil HMOs and fatcat executives on the opposite, creates the worst sort of caricature of reality. Keep your ears open for insightful, constructive critics, but by all means oppose the doomsayers at every turn.

Good healthcare and good business are far from mutually exclusive propositions. Every single American will benefit from, and each has a featured role to play in, a suitably compassionate but responsibly cost-effective healthcare delivery system. The term *"managed care"* elegantly poses the paradox; the manifold arts and sciences of medical caring can be managed like so many businesses, even though healthcare involves a unique human endeavor carried out by entirely unbusinesslike motives, missions, and means. In fact the surest way to reap cost savings is to ensure easy access to just the right healthcare services, even for the healthy, and to manage the timely provision of the highest quality medical care whenever preventive measures fail. Few would challenge these core managed care ideals, and so it is these ideals that must guide our every step forward.

MIND THE GAP

In my eyes, the most prominent feature on the managed-care landscape today is the canyon between perceptions and actualities, promises, and likelihoods. First we need to fix every suspect delivery mechanism and every managed-care technique that might be broken, then we can concentrate on winning more dues-paying converts and achieving the broadest possible participation in the best health plans. Only a fully covered citizenry can sustain managed care's promising trajectory from a shifting cluster of members-only enterprises into a reliable, communitywide system of competitive but cooperative payors and providers who are jointly and severally responsible for monitoring, managing, and improving population health.

The number of citizens in the United States with absolutely no health insurance stands at 40 million and rising! Governments, employers, and the healthcare industry must somehow corral the staggering multitudes who remain uninsurable or stubbornly uninsured. Surely any state-licensed health plan ought to be more than glad to offer some proportion of coverage *pro bono publico,* volunteering to cover one uninsurable life for, say, every dozen paying members. When a plan insists on keeping a strictly business relationship with the community, the community must insist otherwise. Welcome to the battlefront. If far too many remain uncovered, the healthcare wars will rage on and on, revolutionary or civil, hot or cold. Someday soon the frantic and, too often, senseless buying and selling of healthcare interests and enterprises must slacken. Someday soon the pinwheel must come to rest.

We would all do much better to focus on defeating the common enemies of ignorance, disease, pain, and death. My enemy's enemy is my friend. At the end of the day, it is once again the healing mission that must remain top priority and the critical patient-physician relationship that must remain inviolable. For the managed-care community, the noblest call is to support and answer the changing needs of valued members and providers. Please remember that only the free exchange of intellectual capital through advanced information technology and case management techniques, all with a sharp eye toward better health outcomes, will keep managed care moving in the right direction.

In pursuing this course, we must especially be careful to distinguish market maturation from market enlightenment. Any managed healthcare community can grow older, but can yours also manage to grow a little wiser each year? I have witnessed the Canadian and British healthcare systems when they were swept up in the excitement of reform, only to hear the sighs of disappointment years afterward. Other nations' hard lessons are difficult, if not impossible, to translate for the States today. We are finding our own way, of course, and learning plenty by home-grown examples and a healthy dose of trial and error. If nothing else, my expatriations and repatriations have been a study in how quickly such a vital reform movement can get sidetracked. Governments can become inflexible and uncreative, and so can today's so-called free market, if we are not vigilant in our stewardship of change.

The truly lasting changes will arrive but in the fullness of time. And, yes, things might get a whole lot worse before they get better. Some argue that the healthcare system wants to be a fragmented mess. Well, science tells us the human body wants to be a sphere, too, but most specimens outrun that universal rule and embrace the particular, fitter alternative. Once the national healthcare marketplace really opens up, the Profit Motive and a host of equally seductive natural laws such as the bell curve, the 80/20 rule, diminishing returns, averages, supply and demand, and thermodynamics may rule the day. Still, between that moment I wrote these words and this moment you are reading them, the more resonant public health events have transpired not in a reactionary industry that suffers every political season, legislative gridlock, stock market adjustment, and bad public relations piece, but in a universe where the force of momentum equals mass times acceleration. The very bulk of our healthcare economy, our collective will to reduce costs and improve quality, and the swiftness of profound change virtually ensure that we will follow this vector toward a wholly manageable system of population health.

Precisely how we can enact such an inspiring vision is the pressing matter. All we can do is our level best, knowing that managed care offers by far the brightest hope for controlling healthcare costs without compromising on clinical quality. So as the pinwheel blows, where the index points, we go.

I hope this book has helped you better understand your market and given you a guide to map your future. I would love to hear from you real stories from the trenches as you move from managed care lite to heavy. Please send them via e-mail to DennisPatterson1@Compuserve.com.

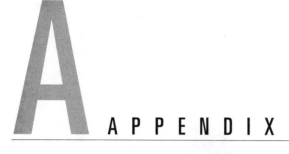

APPENDIX

Extra Pie Workcharts
for Quick Indexing

Patient Managed-Care Incentives

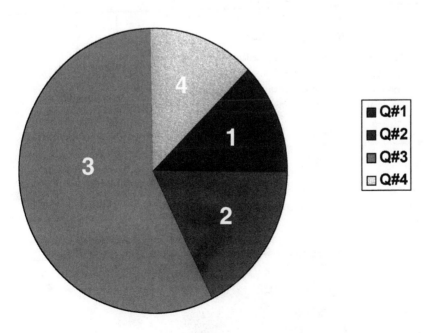

Q#1 No health insurance: leave slice blank for % uninsured

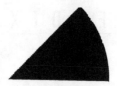

Q#2 Insurance combinations of
- Insured with deductible under $100: blacken ⅓ of slice
- Insured with deductible/copayment $100-$200
- Insured with deductible/copayment above $200: blacken entire slice

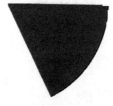

Q#3 Financial incentives
- No financial incentives: leave pie slice blank
- Financial incentive to use restricted panels (1%-10%)
- Financial incentive to use restricted panels (10%-29%)
- Financial incentive to use restricted panels (30%-99%): blacken entire slice

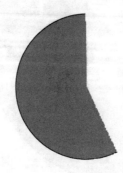

Q#4 Panel restrictions

- No restrictions: leave pie slice blank
- Restricted panel for primary care
- Restricted panel for all medical care
- Restricted panel for all healthcare (mental health, drug abuse, optometrist, diagnostic test, pharmaceuticals): blacken entire slice

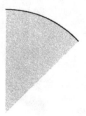

In 1993, using its best SWAG, The Institute for the Future shaded the patient managed-care incentives pie as follows:

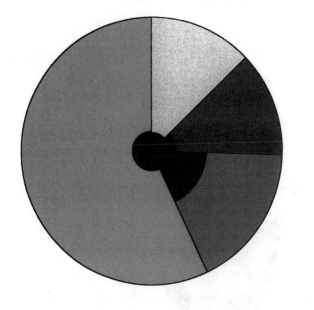

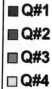

Enrollee Provider Panel Restrictions

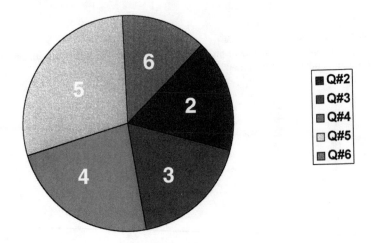

Q#1 No restrictions: do not record

Q#2 Network, 10% or less copayment to go outside:

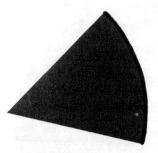

Q#3 Network, 11% or more copayment to go outside:

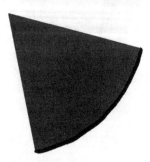

Q#4 Network with gatekeeper, up to 29% or more copayment:

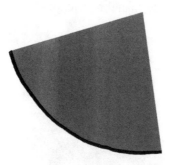

Q#5 Network with gatekeeper, 30% or more copayment:

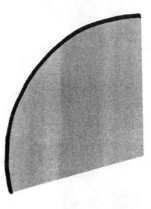

Q#6 Closed panel without point-of-service:

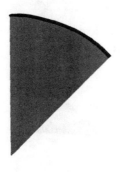

In 1993, The Institute for the Future made the following baseline estimates for enrollee provider panel restrictions.

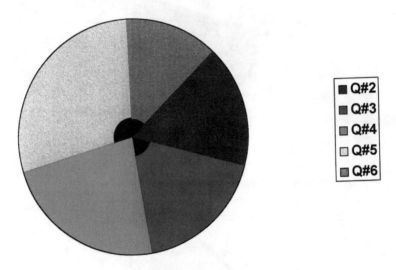

Q#1 No restrictions on prescribing: do not record

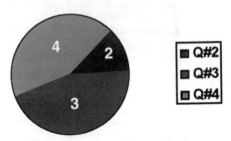

Q#2 No review or restricted formulary—shade % of pie slice that has some restriction

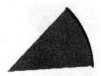

Q#3 Pharmacist review and formulary

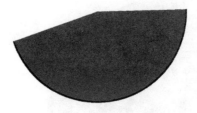

Q#4 Medical director review and use of formulary

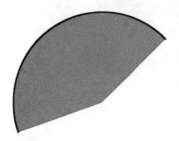

In 1993, The Institute for the Future estimated the use of the process management of pharmaceuticals technique as follows:

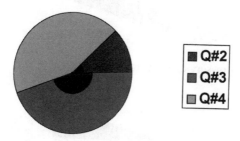

Q#1 Unmanaged fee-for-service: do not record

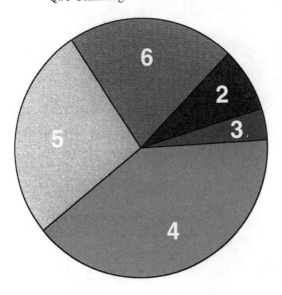

■	Q#2
■	Q#3
■	Q#4
▢	Q#5
■	Q#6

Q#2 Discounted fee-for-service

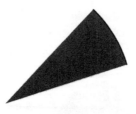

Q#3 Fee-for-service with risk pools

Q#4 Primary care physicians are capitated

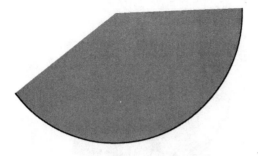

Q#5 Specialists are capitated

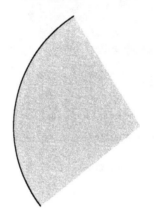

Q#6 Global capitation

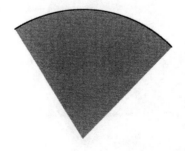

In 1993, The Institute for the Future estimated the use of the physician financial structures technique as follows:

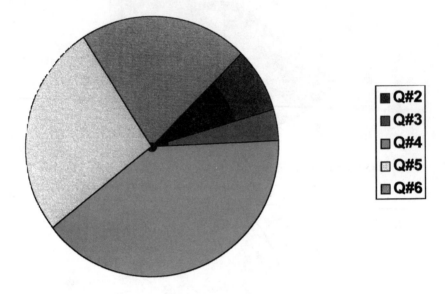

Medical Process Management of Physicians

Q#1 No review: do not record

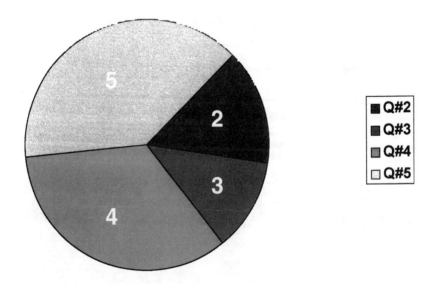

Q#2 Light utilization review (retroactive review)

Q#3 Light process management (prior authorization)

Q#4 Heavy process management (prior and concurrent reviews)

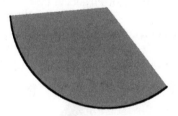

Q#5 Cultural controls (including heavy process management)

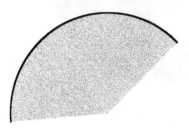

In 1993, The Institute for the Future estimated the use of a medical process management of physicians technique as follows:

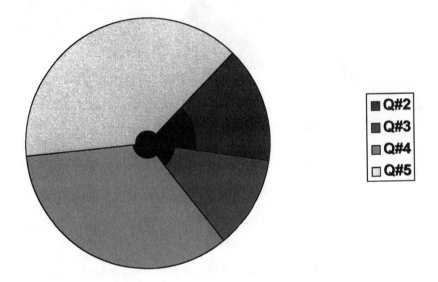

Organizational Structure of Physician Practice Setting

Q#1 Independent practice, one or two doctors: do not record

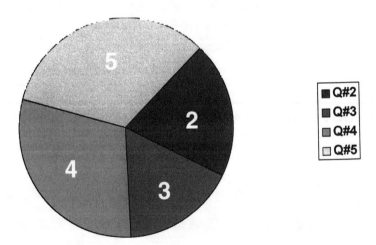

Q#2 Single-specialty group or IPA practice

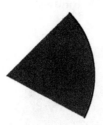

Q#3 Small multispecialty group or IPA practice

Q#4 Medium multispecialty group or IPA practice

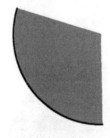

Q#5 Large multispecialty group

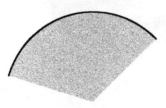

In 1993, The Institute for the Future estimated the organizational structure of physician practice setting as follows:

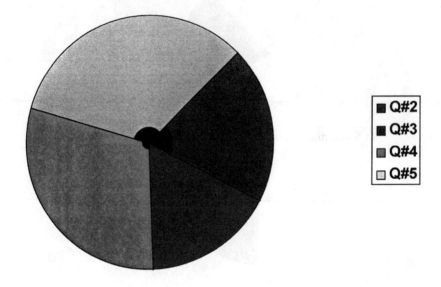

Physician Referral Access

Q#1 No restrictions: do not record

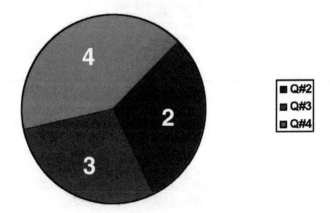

Q#2 Preferred Provider Organization (PPO)(general restrictions)

Q#3 Closed panel restrictions (some specialties)

Q#4 Closed panel restrictions (all specialties)

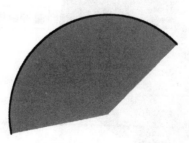

In 1993, The Institute for the Future estimated the restriction of physician referral access as follows:

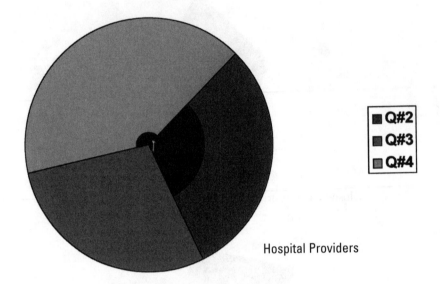

Hospital Providers

Medical Risk Population

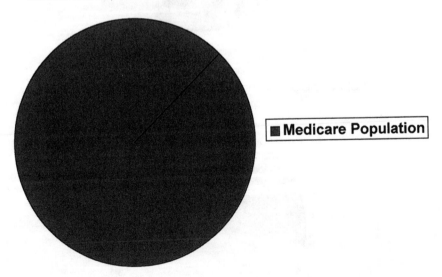

Medicare Population

In 1993, The Institute for the Future estimated the Medicare population to be as follows:

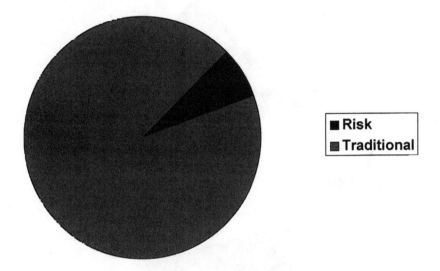

Hospital Medical Process Management

Q#1 No restrictions: do not record

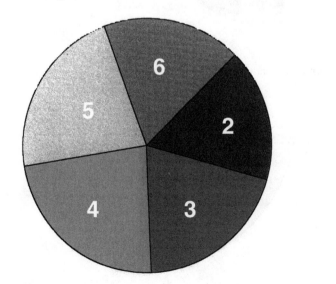
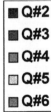

Q#2 Preadmission certification (only)

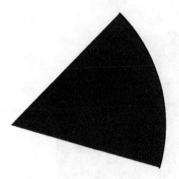

Q#3 Discharge planning

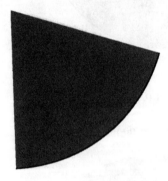

Q#4 Concurrent utilization review (case management)

Q#5 Detailed practice guidelines or critical pathways

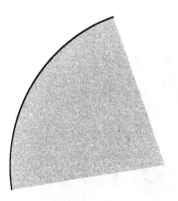

Q#6 Clinical continuous quality improvement/total quality management

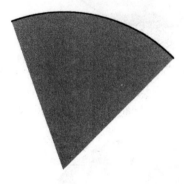

In 1993, The Institute for the Future estimated the use of hospital medical-process management as follows:

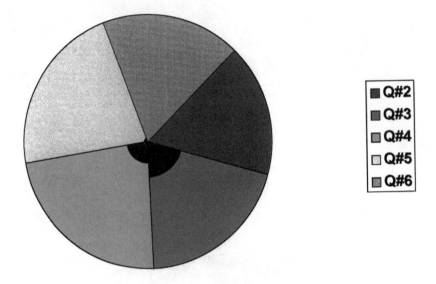

Risk Sharing Among Hospitals, Physicians, and Payors

Q#1 Payor (carrier) bears full risk: do not record

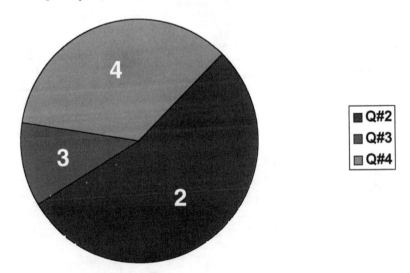

Q#2 Payor shares risk with physician

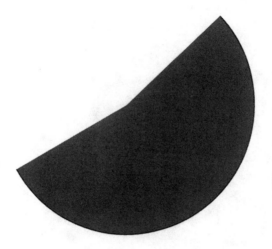

Q#3 Payor shares risk with hospital

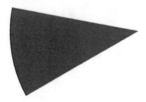

Q#4 Shared risk among payor, hospital, and physicians

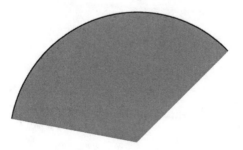

In 1993, The Institute of the Future estimated very little risk sharing among providers, as follows:

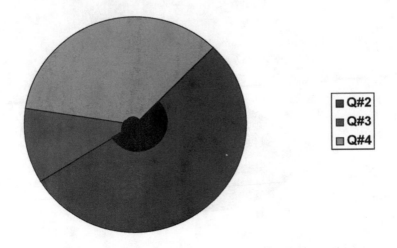

APPENDIX

Baseline Index Scales, Weights, and Scoring

The quick indexing exercise presented in Chapter 5, complete with the extra pie workcharts included in Appendix A, will suffice for those who simply want a clearer view of their managed-care marketplaces at-a-glance. For those who desire and are capable of employing a more rigorous quantitative method, this appendix presents the metrics used by the architects of the managed-care index.

Figure B–1 illustrates the overall conceptual framework behind the managed-care index. In essence, the index tracks the telltale signs of managed-care evolution (financial incentives, micromanagement, integration of medicine, provider panel restrictions, and acceptance) exhibited by all major healthcare system participants, both users (patients, enrollees) and providers (physicians, hospitals, pharmacies). This matrix shows the measurable, aggregate managed-care activities of the main participants in our healthcare system. Shaded areas denote the managed-care indicators for which the index incorporates a broad range of user and provider data. Figure B–2, the Managed-Care Fishbone diagram, then shows how these measures figure in the calculation of index scores.

The following sections detail the scale of activities we considered, possible survey questions, and original Institute for the Future baseline estimates that helped us calibrate our model and, ultimately, design and refine the index.

FIGURE B–1

The Managed-Care Index:
Conceptual Framework, Activities of System Participants

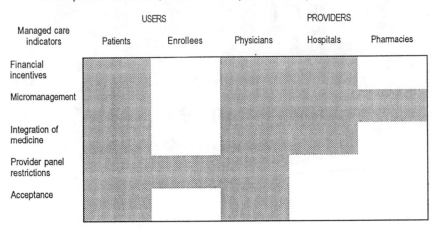

Patient Managed-Care Incentives

This indicator concerns the incentives (and disincentives) that influence the behavior of patients and enrollees. The index categorizes patient managed-care incentives along the following scale, in ascending order from zero managed care to managed-care lite to fully managed care:

- No Health insurance;
- Insured
  —with no access restrictions; no or small ($100 and under) deductible/co-pay;
  —with premium sharing; and
  —with deductible/co-payment above $100 to preset limit.
- Lite managed care, featuring use of insurance subject to
  —prehospital certification;
  —incentives for prehospital testing;
  —utilization review;
  —higher reimbursement at birthing center;
  —higher reimbursement for generic drugs;
  —limited reimbursement for weekend nonemergency hospital admission;

F I G U R E   B – 2

The Managed-Care Index "Fishbone"

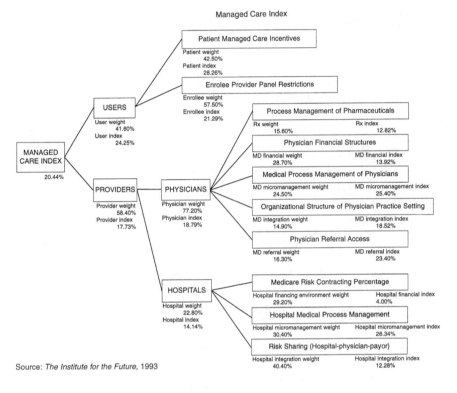

Source: *The Institute for the Future,* 1993

—separate deductible for hospital admission; and

—higher reimbursement for mail-order drugs.

- Financial incentives to use restricted panel
    —savings from 1% to 10%;
    —savings from 11% to 20%; and
    —savings greater than 21%.
- Restricted panel for all primary care;
- Restricted panel for all medical care; and
- Restricted panel for all healthcare, including mental health, drug abuse, optometry, and other needs such as diagnostic tests and pharmaceuticals.

A consumer survey, featuring at least the following questions, can be used to gather the required data.

- Do you have health insurance?
- Who provides you with your health insurance (Medicare, employer, spouse, self)?
- For what portion of the health insurance premiums are you responsible (all, some, or none)? If some, how much do you pay per month ($0 to $50, $50 to $100, $100 +)?
- What is the size of your deductible and co-payments? What is your maximum charge per year?
- Is your insurance coverage subject to any of the following conditions?
  —prehospital certification
  —incentives for prehospital testing
  —utilization review
  —higher reimbursement at birthing center
  —higher reimbursement for generic drugs
  —limited reimbursement for weekend nonemergency hospital admission
  —separate deductible for hospital admission
  —higher reimbursement for mail-order drugs
- Do you have a financial incentive to use a restricted panel of doctors? How large are your potential savings?
- Do you have a restricted panel for primary care needs only? for specialists? for other health professionals? for diagnostic tests and pharmacy needs? for all health care needs?

Table B–1 shows the baseline estimates for patient managed-care incentives, as devised by The Institute for the Future in 1993.

Enrollee Provider Panel Restrictions

This indicator concerns the incentives (and disincentives) that influence patients' and enrollees' choice of physicians. The index categorizes patient managed-care incentives along the following scale, in ascending order from zero managed care to managed-care lite to fully managed care:

- No restrictions, fee-for-service;
- Preferred provider organization, large panel (95% of doctors);
- Gatekeeper, restricted direct access to specialists;

TABLE B-1

Patient Managed-Care Incentives
Baseline Estimates, 1993

Scale	Share of Total Population, %
No health insurance	13
Insured	
—with no access restrictions; no or small ($100 and under) deductible/co-pay	4
—with deductible/co-payment above $100 to preset limit	8
Lite managed care, featuring use of insurance subject to	
—prehospital certification	
—incentives for prehospital testing	
—utilization review	
—higher reimbursement at birthing center	
—higher reimbursement for generic drugs	
—limited reimbursement for weekend nonemergency admission	
—separate deductible for hospital admission	
—higher reimbursement for mail-order drugs	
Share with at least two from the above list	22
Share with at least four from the above list	14
Share with at least six from the above list	6
Financial incentives to use restricted panel	
—savings from 1% to 10%	5
—savings from 11% to 20%	5
—savings greater than 21%	5
Restricted panel for all primary care	9
Restricted panel for all medical care	6
Restricted panel for all healthcare	3

Source: *The Institute for the Future,* 1993

- Closed panel with point-of-service option (30% of doctors); and
- Closed panel without point-of-service (one medical group).

The enrollee data gathered here is available from several excellent national sources, including the American Association of Health Plans, InterStudy, and the Health Insurance Association of America.

Table B–2 shows the baseline estimates for enrollee provider panel restrictions, as devised by The Institute for the Future in 1993.

TABLE B-2

Enrollee Provider Panel Restrictions
Baseline Estimates, 1993

Scale	Share of Total Enrollee Population, %
No restrictions	65
PPO large panel	16
Gatekeeper	1
Closed panel with point-of-service	6
Closed panel without point-of-service	12

Source: *The Institute for the Future,* 1993

Physician Financial Structures

This indicator concerns the financial incentives (and disincentives) that influence the behavior of physicians. The index categorizes physician financial structures along the following scale, in ascending order from zero managed care to managed-care lite to fully managed care:

- Unmanaged fee-for-service;
- Discounted fee-for-service;
- Fee-for-service with risk pool withhold;
- Capitation; and
- Salary.

A physician survey, featuring at least the following questions, can be used to gather the required data.

- What percentage of your patients originate from each of the financial structures listed above?
- What portion of your practice revenues does each of these financial structures represent?

Table B–3 shows the baseline estimates for physician financial structures, as devised by The Institute for the Future in 1993.

TABLE B-3

Physician Financial Structures
Baseline Estimates, 1993

Scale	Patients, %	Revenues, %
Unmanaged fee-for-service	5	10
Discounted fee-for-service	45	25
Fee-for-service with risk pool	10	10
Capitation	10	8
Salary	5	7

Source: *The Institute for the Future*, 1993

Medical Process Management of Physicians

This indicator concerns the medical micromanagement of physicians using various utilization review and cultural controls. The index categorizes medical process management of physicians along the following scale, in ascending order from zero managed care to managed-care lite to fully managed care:

- No review;
- Light utilization review controls (score of 1 to 6);
- Heavy utilization review controls (score of 6 to 13); and
- "Cultural" controls (score of 13 to 22).

The scores above are based on the following point system:

- Light utilization review, each worth 1 point
  —precertification for hospitalization
  —precertification for testing or office procedures
  —precertification for day surgery
  —postcare feedback on individual claims
- Heavy utilization review, each worth 2 points
  —enforced formulary
  —enforced practice guidelines
  —clinical profiling

- Cultural controls, each worth 3 points
  —economic profiling
  —feedback on clinical profiling
  —feedback on economic profiling
  —formal peer review

A physician survey, featuring at least the following questions, can be used to gather the required data.

- What percentage of your patients are subject to each of the controls listed above?
- Which of these controls are you subject to for at least half of your patients?
- For each control to which you are subject, does an external payor or someone in your own organization perform the review?

Table B–4 shows the baseline estimates for medical process management of physicians, as devised by The Institute for the Future in 1993.

Organizational Structure of Physician Practice Setting

This indicator concerns the physician group size and level of integration. The index categorizes the organizational structure of physician practice settings along the following scale, in ascending order from zero managed care to managed-care lite to fully managed care:

- Independent practice, one or two doctors;
- Single-specialty group practice;
- Small multispecialty group practice;

TABLE B–4

Medical Process Management of Physicians
Baseline Estimates, 1993

Scale	Physicians, %
No review	5
Light UR controls	33
Heavy UR controls	12
"Cultural" controls	10

Source: *The Institute for the Future,* 1993

- Medium multispecialty group practice;
- Large multispecialty group practice; and
- Integrated system (continuum of care).

A physician survey, featuring at least the following questions, can be used to gather the required data.

- Do you practice solo or in a group? How many doctors are in the group?
- Is your group single- or multispecialty? If multispecialty, what percentage of your group practice is primary care?
- Are you part of an integrated medical system?
- Does your organization deliver mental healthcare? home healthcare? long-term care?

Table B–5 shows the baseline estimates for organization structure of physician practice settings, as devised by The Institute for the Future in 1993.

Physician Referral Access

This indicator concerns the restrictions placed on physicians to refer patients and enrollees to other physicians. The index categorizes physician referral access along the following scale, in ascending order from zero managed care to managed-care lite to fully managed care:

TABLE B–5

Organization Structure of Physician Practice Settings
Baseline Estimates, 1993

Scale	Physicians, %
Independent practice	60.0
Single-specialty group practice	18.6
Small multispecialty group practice	4.4
Medium multispecialty group practice	4.6
Large multispecialty group practice	9.4
Integrated system (continuum of care)	3.0

Source: *The Institute for the Future*, 1993

- No restrictions;
- Preferred provider organization, general restrictions; and
- Health maintenance organization, closed-panel restrictions.

A physician survey, featuring at least the following questions, can be used to gather the required data.

- What percentage of your patients belong to plans that have
  —no referral restrictions?
  —referral restrictions for a wide range of physicians (PPO type)?
  —restrictions to certain specialists or for tests?
  —referral to closed panel of physicians only?

Table B–6 shows the baseline estimates for physician referral access, as devised by The Institute for the Future in 1993.

Medicare Risk Contracting Percentage

This indicator concerns the penetration of managed care into a market's Medicare population. The index scale for Medicare risk contracting, figured on a strict percentage basis using HCFA data, will surely evolve as the federal government moves more and more of the Medicare population into managed-care products.

Hospital Financial Incentives

This indicator concerns the incentives for physicians to reduce hospital admissions. The index categorizes hospital financial incentives along the following scale, in ascending order from zero managed care to managed-care lite to fully managed care:

TABLE B – 6

Physician Referral Access
Baseline Estimates, 1993

Scale	Patients, %
No restrictions	40
PPO, general restrictions	45
HMO, closed-panel restrictions	15

Source: *The Institute for the Future,* 1993

- Fee-for-service;
- Discounted fee-for-service;
- Per diem;
- Diagnosis-related group;
- Capitation; and
- Budget (global).

A physician survey, featuring at least the following questions, can be used to gather the required data.

- Do you have incentives to reduce your hospital admissions?
- If so, do the incentives include
  —capitation?
  —withholds?
  —withholds plus bonuses?
  —other (please specify)?

Table B–7 shows the baseline estimates for hospital financial incentives, as devised by The Institute for the Future in 1993.

Hospital Medical Process Management

This indicator concerns the sophistication hospitals exhibit in micro-managing core medical processes for optimum efficiency and effective-ness. The index categorizes hospital medical process management along

TABLE B–7

Hospital Financial Incentives
Baseline Estimates, 1993

Scale	Revenues, %
Fee-for-service	5
Discounted fee-for-service	40
Per diem	—
DRG	40
Capitation	—
Budget (global)	—

Source: *The Institute for the Future,* 1993

the following scale, in ascending order from zero managed care to managed-care lite to fully managed care:

- Preadmission certification;
- Discharge planning, by payor;
- Discharge planning, by hospital;
- Concurrent utilization review (case management); and
- Detailed practice guidelines or critical pathways.

A physician survey, featuring at least the following questions, can be used to gather the required data.

- Do you admit to hospitals?
- If so, what percentage of your patients are subject to
  —preadmission certification?
  —discharge planning, by payor?
  —discharge planning, by hospital?
  —concurrent utilization review (case management)?
  —detailed practice guidelines or critical pathways?

Hospital Integration of Medicine

This indicator concerns the closeness of the affiliation between hospitals and physicians. The index categorizes hospital integration of medicine along the following scale, in ascending order from zero managed care to managed-care lite to fully managed care:

- No integration;
- Hospital-physician alliance, such as joint foundation or joint equity models;
- Salaried physicians; and
- Group model HMO.

A physician survey, featuring at least the following questions, can be used to gather the required data.

- Do you have a relationship with one or more hospitals?
- If so, can that relationship(s) be characterized as
  —occasional admitting privileges to hospital(s)?
  —split admissions between or among hospitals?
  —exclusive admitting privileges to hospital(s)?

—member of an independent practice association affiliated with hospital(s)?

—member of a formal physician-hospital organization?

—member of a group in an integrated model (such as a foundation model)?

—employee of hospital (if so, are you a radiologist? anesthesiologist? pathologist?)?

Process Management of Pharmaceuticals

This indicator concerns the micromanagement of pharmaceutical prescriptions and therapy. The index categorizes process management of pharmaceuticals along the following scale, in ascending order from zero managed care to managed-care lite to fully managed care:

- No restrictions on prescribing;
- Physician subject to one or more of the following, though with no formal enforcement mechanism;
  —generic substitution policies
  —mail-order policies for maintenance drugs
  —nonrestrictive formularies
- Physician also subject to one or more of the following, though with no formal enforcement mechanism;
  —restrictive formularies
  —practice guidelines with step therapy policies
- Physician subject to one or more of the following, with enforcement by pharmacists at the point of dispensing;
  —generic substitution policies
  —mail-order policies for maintenance drugs
  —nonrestrictive formularies
- Physician also subject to one or more of the following, with enforcement by pharmacists at the point of dispensing;
  —restrictive formularies
  —practice guidelines with step therapy policies
- Physician subject to one or more of the following, with immediate enforcement at the point of prescribing;
  —generic substitution policies
  —mail-order policies for maintenance drugs
  —nonrestrictive formularies

■ Physician also subject to one or more of the following, with immediate enforcement at the point of prescribing

—restrictive formularies

—practice guidelines with step therapy policies.

A physician survey instrument, perhaps in the form of a matrix like the one shown in Table B–8, can best gather information about the prescription policies and enforcements listed above.

Table B–9 shows the baseline estimates for process management of pharmaceuticals, as devised by The Institute for the Future in 1993.

Risk Sharing Among Hospitals, Physicians, and Payors

This indicator concerns the extent to which the different blades of the pinwheel share business and clinical risk with other blades. The index categorizes risk sharing along the following scale, in ascending

TABLE B–8

Process Management of Pharmaceuticals
Physician Survey Matrix

	Policy Exists, No Formal Enforcement	Enforcement at Point of Dispensing (Pharmacist Mediates)	Enforcement at Point of Prescribing (Physician Directly Linked)
Generic substitution			
Mail-order policy for maintenance drugs			
Nonrestrictive formulary			
Restrictive formulary			
Practice guidelines with step therapy policy			

TABLE B-9

Process Management of Pharmaceuticals
Baseline Estimates, 1993

Scale	Physicians, %
No restrictions on prescribing	44
One or more of following, no formal enforcement —generic substitution policies —mail-order policies for maintenance drugs —nonrestrictive formularies	3
Also one or more of following, no formal enforcement —restrictive formularies —practice guidelines with step therapy policies	17
One or more of following, pharmacists enforce at dispensing —generic substitution policies —mail-order policies for maintenance drugs —nonrestrictive formularies	15
Also one or more of following, pharmacists enforce at dispensing —restrictive formularies —practice guidelines with step therapy policies	19
One or more of following, enforced at point of prescribing —generic substitution policies —mail-order policies for maintenance drugs —nonrestrictive formularies	1
Also one or more of following, enforced at point of prescribing —restrictive formularies —practice guidelines with step therapy policies	1

Source: *The Institute for the Future*, 1993

order from zero managed care to managed-care lite to fully managed care:

- Payor (carrier) bears full risk;
- Payor shares risk with physicians;
- Payor shares risk with hospital; and
- Shared risk between payor, physician, and hospital.

Managed-care indexers may need to combine surveys of payors, physicians, and hospitals with a careful, objective study to get a fix on marketplace sharing of risk.

TABLE B-10

Physician Acceptance
Baseline Estimates, 1993

Scale	Physicians, %
Strongly oppose	30
Begrudgingly accept	60
Strongly favor	10

Source: *The Institute for the Future,* 1993

Patient Acceptance

This indicator is really nothing more than a patient satisfaction survey. The index categorizes patient acceptance of managed care according to the following scale:

- Very dissatisfied;
- Somewhat dissatisfied;
- Somewhat satisfied; or
- Very satisfied.

A straightforward survey question might ask, How do you feel about the healthcare services you and your family have used in the last few years?

Physician Acceptance

The index categorizes physician acceptance of managed care according to the following scale:

- Strongly oppose;
- Begrudgingly accept; or
- Strongly favor.

A straightforward survey question might ask: In recent years, most doctors have seen many of their patients move into managed-care health plans. How do you feel about this trend? Do you strongly oppose, begrudgingly accept, or strongly favor it?

Table B–10 shows the baseline estimates for physician acceptance, as devised by The Institute for the Future in 1993.

ABOUT THE AUTHOR

Dennis J. Patterson is a Consultant in healthcare in Southern California. His career has been an intensive study in comparative national healthcare systems and advanced organizational management, design, and redesign. Educated and trained in the United States, Mr. Patterson spent the 1970s in Canada as a hospital administrator at large teaching institutions. In the 1980s he entered management consulting, first directing his own consulting firm and then joining Ernst & Whinney's midwest practice in Chicago. He was called to Ernst & Young's London office, where he served as partner in charge of healthcare for the United Kingdom, and later to Los Angeles, where he turned his attention exclusively toward managed-care organizations. For three years he was chief executive officer of FHP International Consulting Group, formerly a subsidiary of FHP International Corporation, then California's fourth largest HMO. Mr. Patterson has served as a trustee of George Washington University Medical Center and of the California School of Professional Psychology. He publishes and speaks throughout the world on a wide variety of healthcare and business topics and has consulted in Canada, Germany, Iceland, Mexico, Spain, the United Kingdom, and the United States.

INDEX